Current Approaches The Problem of Recurrent Abdominal Pain

Edited by
A Dawson & S W Parker

**duphar
medical relations**

First published 1989

ISBN 1-870678-10-9

Printed in Great Britain by
Inprint (Litho) Ltd., Southampton.

CLINICAL FEATURES OF THE IRRITABLE BOWEL SYNDROME

K Heaton
Reader in Medicine
Bristol Royal Infirmary

Prevalence

We are currently conducting a survey in Bristol to look at the prevalence of functional intestinal symptoms. The approach is new in that we are collecting data from a sample drawn at random from the general population. Preliminary results concerning abdominal pain from the first 492 people surveyed are shown below.

Table 1: Prevalence of abdominal pain in a stratified random sample of men aged 40-69 and woman aged 20-69.

	Males (=204)	Females (=288)
Experienced abdominal pain in past 12 months	54	102
Lower abdominal pain on more than 6 days (other than dysmenorrhoea)	15 (7%)	58 (20%)
Lower abdominal pain often or always relieved by defaecation:	8 (4%)	28 (10%)

On the basis of these findings it is apparent that 10% of the women questioned and 4% of the men admit to symptoms which a GP or gastroenterologist would diagnose as irritable bowel syndrome or spastic colon. The true prevalence of the condition is probably nearer to 15% of the population, given that the pain of IBS is not always in the lower abdomen, and is not relieved by defaecation in every case.

Diagnosis

Despite being such a common syndrome, perhaps even the commonest of all named syndromes, it remains the least confidently diagnosed. There are several reasons. Not all doctors are aware of the protean nature of the syndrome. Symptoms are multiple and occur in endlessly varying combinations. The task of history - taking is a lengthy and involved one if all the relevant details are to be identified. It requires tact and sensitivity to elicit information about functions of the body which people find shameful or disgusting and which, furthermore, lack a familiar and accurate vocabulary.

Textbook teaching itself is a source of diagnostic hesitation and anxiety. The conventional definition of irritable bowel syndrome refers to adominal pain and/or altered bowel habit due to changes in colonic motility and explains the lack of confidence of so many doctors in making a diagnosis of IBS. Much unnecessary investigation is involved and the doctor constantly harbours some anxiety about missing significant pathology.

Definitions

The word "syndrome" comes from the Greek expression meaning, simply, "concurrence" and a medical dictionary definition would be of a "symptom complex" . This being so, our definition of IBS should surely concentrate on the ways symptoms cluster together to produce the IBS and not on the negative and unhelpful "absence of organic disease" . A better definition might run something like this:

A variable but characteristic combination of symptoms attributable to the intestines, especially abdominal or periabdominal pain, bloating, distension and symptoms of disturbed defaecation.

An international working party has been set up to agree criteria for diagnosis and their recommended definition is similar to this one. Eventually, we will recognise sub-types of the disease.

Symptoms of Disturbed Defaecation

These are the most characteristic symptoms and, at the same time, the ones the patient finds it most difficult to talk about. To elicit these symptoms needs all the skills of the doctor.They include:

Urgent calls to stool
More frequent calls to stool   } symptoms of an irritable
Feelings of incomplete evacuation   rectum or inappropriate
Feelings of needing to strain   rectal signals
Stools reduced in size
Changes in consistency and shape of stools
Loss of normal call to stool
Less regular calls to stool

Characteristics of Pain in IBS

Pain is the symptom most likely to precipitate a consultation in the patient with IBS. There are certain characteristics shared by IBS pain sufferers. Firstly, the pain is often experienced in several places. This is not well described in textbooks but is common knowledge to experienced gastroenterologists. We have documented this quite clearly in over 30 patients who were asked to keep daily symptom diaries for 31 days. Many describe multiple pains which vary in type, duration and intensity and this I regard as one of the hallmarks of functional pain as opposed to organic pain which tends to be relatively stereotyped. Furthermore, the pain in IBS is often poorly localised and can even be generalised which, again, is unlike organic pain. Colonic pain is often at its worst an hour or two after a meal and stress is sometimes, but not very often, a recognised provoking factor.

The symptom of pain relief on defaecation is the most helpful aspect of IBS pain because it points specifically to the lower bowel as the source of pain. In my experience 75-80% of patients admit to relief with defaecation. Changes in stool frequency and form at times of pain also link pain with the bowel. The association between pain and defaecation enables a confident diagnosis of intestinal pain to be made.

Sites of Pain

Lower abdominal pain is frequently but by no means exclusively reported. The wide distribution of pain in IBS has given rise to considerable speculation about the origin of the pain but there is persuasive evidence from studies involving balloon dilatation at various sites in the colon (1) that distension at one location is able to provoke pain in diverse and varying sites of the abdomen. Often the induced pains replicated the pains suffered by patients during episodes of IBS. In some patients in whom the original pain was not reproduced by balloon dilatation of the colon, typical IBS pain could be reproduced by balloon dilatation in other sites in the gastrointestinal tract including oesophagus and small intestine. (2)

Further evidence implicating abnormal intestinal function in the IBS comes from pressure recordings made from the lower bowel. In IBS patients in whom continuous intrasigmoid and intrarectal pressure is measured a clear correlation can sometimes be seen between peak intestinal pressures and pain, which seems to support the notion, widely believed, that it is spasm of the gut which causes pain. This is not necessarily so. A contraction which holds up the onwards movement of bowel contents can produce distension proximally and it may be the distension rather than the contraction which produces pain. In fact, pressures are not consistently higher in IBS patients. Nobody has been able to unequivocally distinguish IBS sufferers from normals on the basis of colon motility alone. Therefore, the possibility is still very much alive that the gut of the IBS sufferer is more sensitive than normal rather than more active than normal.

Indeed, there is good evidence to support such a hypothesis. Richie distended balloons in the sigmoid colon and found that most normal subjects felt pain at a volume of 120 ml or more whereas IBS patients usually reported pain at 60 ml or less.(3) There seems to be increased sensitivity of other lower abdominal organs in IBS patients. Dyspareunia, in particular, is common as are symptoms of disturbed micturition which parallel the symptoms of disturbed defaecation .(4) So it is, perhaps, not just the bowel which is irritable in these patients but sometimes the bladder and other organs as well.

Whorwell's IBS patient sample also admitted to many more non-specific symptoms and psychoneurotic symptoms than the normal controls, which could be interpreted as showing that IBS patients are neurotic and hypochondriacal. Caution should be exercised, however, in generalising the results of a small select group of patients with entrenched symptoms who had been referred to a consultant with a special interest in IBS. The experiences of this particularly difficult group of patients may well not be representative of all the IBS sufferers who attend GPs, let alone the ones who never present to a doctor at all. In our own survey in Bristol (5) the most striking statistic was that 80% of people admitting to spastic colon symptoms had never consulted their doctor about the problem. It is essential to distinguish between the causes of the syndrome on one hand and the factors which determine who seeks help for their symptoms on the other.

Aetiological Factors

These include dietary changes, constipation, travel, food intolerance and stress. The main factors leading to treatment seeking are probably anxiety, depression and learned illness behaviour but presumably severe symptoms, especially pain, are more likely to be reported than mild symptoms. (6)

References

1. Swarbrick ET, Hegarty JE, Bat L, Williams CB, Dawson AM. Site of pain from the irritable bowel. *Lancet* 1980; 2: 443-6.

2. Moriarty KJ, Dawson AM. Functional abdominal pain: further evidence that whole gut is affected. *Br Med J* 1982; 284: 1670-2.

3. Ritchie J. Pain from distension of the pelvic colon by inflating a balloon in the irritable bowel syndrome. *Gut* 1973; 14: 125-32.

4. Whorwell PJ, McCallum M, Creed FH, et al. Non-colonic features of irritable bowel syndrome. *Gut* 1986; 27: 37-40.

5. Thompson WG, Heaton KW. Functional bowel disorders in apparently healthy people. *Gastroenterol* 1980; 79: 283-8.

6. Drossman DA, McMee DC, Sandler RS, et al. Psychosocial factors in irritable bowel syndrome. A multi-variate study. *Gastroenterol* 1987; 92: 1374.

Discussion

Moriarty: You talk about "the irritable bowel syndrome" and others refer to " the irritable gut". Some of us prefer the expression "functional gastrointestinal disorder" to emphasise that the symptoms can involve the whole gut. What are your thoughts about looking at IBS from a purely symptomatic point of view? This is particularly important when you are dealing with associated symptoms like, for example, a bad taste on the tongue or abdominal distension. This approach has the added advantage that it suggests different treatment approaches which may be appropriate. For example, whilst bran may help those people in whom constipation predominates, it only adds to the problem of the patient whose main complaint is distension or who have frequent loose motions. I put this point to you for your comments because I know you often advocate the use of bran and I feel that it is important in therapeutic trials to dissect out the various subgroups of patients.

Heaton: I agree with everything you have said. I think we have been intellectually lazy in the past about trying to understand individual symptoms. If the complaint is of straining at stool we have too often accepted the patient's word for it that they are constipated, we have not actually asked them to record what type of stool there was. Also, if they have frequent stools, we accept their word that they have diarrhoea; again, we do not record the type of stools that they pass. We now know that a lot of constipation, especially in younger women, is not caused by low stool weight but by a difficulty in relaxing the anal sphincter, such that when they strain to defaecate, the sphincter may even tighten up. We need to be finding what the physiological correlates are for the different symptoms at all the different levels of the gut. There certainly are upper gut symptoms in some of these people if you enquire for them but I thought with the emphasis on lower abdominal pain today, I would by-pass that end of the gut.

Audience: Have you looked at your own group of patients, or those from Richard Harvey, to see whether those who have pain but no bowel disturbance have a different distribution of pain from those patients with bowel disturbance?

Heaton: Yes. We did that with our first survey. (5) A cluster analysis of symptoms showed that indeed the lower abdominal pains clustered with the bloating, the feelings of incomplete evacuation with harder stools and also looser stools than normal. This was a very definite cluster which correlated with what we had previously defined as being typical IBS or spastic colon syndrome. Other upper abdominal pains were associated with less clearly defined clusters. Some of them were post-prandial pains with no bowel features at all or dyspepsia. Other upper abdominal pains were relieved by defaecation and associated with the other rectal symptoms; the distinction was not clear-cut. Functional dyspepsia is a syndrome which I suspect is even less well understood than IBS.

Audience: Is there a group of symptoms which characterise patients who have a spasm of the colon and another group of symptoms typical of distention?

Heaton : No. We have no way of distinguishing what is going on in the patient, whether there is spasm or distension or, indeed, whether it is possible to separate them. Distension may be the inevitable consequence of spasm. The study of gut motility is bedevilled with methodological problems which make interpretation of findings very difficult. The detection and quantification of spasm and distension is still in a very embryonic stage.

DOES SURGERY HAVE A PLACE IN THE MANAGEMENT OF CHRONIC ABDOMINAL PAIN?

J G C Kingham
Consultant Physician
Morriston Hospital Swansea

There are patients with recurrent abdominal pain who have a straightforward, easily diagnosed organic disorder, but they are in the minority. So, what happens to patients who have recurrent pain? This depends on where they are referred to, and referral patterns vary greatly across the country from hospital to hospital depending on local resources. There has been a change over the past 20 years or so with gastroenterology becoming a specialty in its own right so that there are now many more physicians with a special interest in the abdomen than there once were. Even so only about 50% of patient in a representative hospital district will be referred to a physician. The other 50% will be referred to surgical specialties, either general surgeons or perhaps to gynaecologists. Outcomes differ greatly depending on referral which reflects more about differences in the way we are taught and teach those who work with us than it does about abdominal pain. Standard texts discuss the perception of visceral pain in terms of pain maps most of which are derived from sophisticated studies done half a century ago (1,2) where visceral pain was induced in normal subjects by balloon insufflation. If the upper visceral organs were distended (stomach, duodenum, biliary tract) then pain was perceived in the midline in the epigastrium. Visceral pain from the small intestine was perceived in the midline around the umbilicus and from the colon pain was referred to the hypogastrium. Familiar though this may be it must be remembered that this data was derived from normal subjects and not from patients complaining of abdominal pain. The same texts teach that if tenderness is experienced laterally this implies that no longer is one dealing only with visceral pain, but that the parietes are involved. This works well for acute abdominal syndromes, such as appendicitis, cholecystitis and diverticulitis, but the pain map approach really does not seem to work quite so well for chronic abdominal pain.

In the '50s and '60s there were a number of classical papers on the irritable bowel syndrome pointing out that it was a common disorder, that it tended to affect younger age groups, that it affected women more commonly than men and that the diagnosis was unlikely to be made in more than a small proportion (10%) of patients at the time of referral. More notably, up to 30% of these patients with functional abdominal pain had already been operated on inappropriately.(3) Following up a group of 50 patients deemed to have irritable bowel syndrome, produced a pain map showing that the majority of patients did not have their pain in the midline where we are taught to expect that visceral pain should be perceived, but in at least half of the cases the pain was lateralised. Neither was it always where one would expect to find colonic pain, being often reported in the upper abdomen, and 10 of the patients had more than one pain. It's easy to understand how patients who complained of pain in the right hypochondrium, particularly if it radiated round to the back or to the shoulder, were thought to have biliary colic and those with pain in the left upper quadrant were thought to have peptic or pancreatic disease, whilst patients with pain in the right iliac fossa were thought to have ileocaecal or appendiceal disease. Patients with lower pelvic pain might easily be assumed to have a gynaecological disorder. Many of these points are illustrated by a study of 66 patients with so-called intractable functional abdominal pain which was carried out at St. Bartholomew's Hospital (4), 61 of the 66 patients had had a previous hospital consultation for this complaint. 21 had been referred from their primary care physician direct to a gastroenterologist, whilst two-thirds had been referred from another specialist either to a gastroenterologist or to a psychiatrist. 34 of the 66 patients had previously undergone surgery, mainly cholecystectomy, gynaecological procedure or laparotomy. When these patients were psychiatrically assessed the most common form of psychopathology was depression and this diagnosis had by and large been missed all along the line.

Dr Heaton has already referred to Swarbrick's study(5) in which the characteristic pain suffered by patients with irritable bowel syndrome could often be reproduced by insufflating a balloon within the colon. Not only could the abdominal pain be precipitated but so too in many cases could the patient's customary referred pain be reproduced, including the lumber spine, the right shoulder and lower ribs, the loins, sacroiliac region, perineum and thigh. Patients with pain that radiated to the right lower ribs could easily be thought to have biliary tract disease. Pain in the loins in several of these patients had led to mistaken diagnoses of renal tract disease. Pain went down to the sacro-iliac region, to the perineum and the vulva in quite a number of patients, and these patients were thought to have had gynaecological disorders beforehand.

Whorwell (6) found that dyspareunia, bladder symptoms and back pain were extremely common, affecting about 50% of their group of 90 female patients, which was between 4 and 8 times commoner than in a control population of 100 patients. Once again, it is easy to understand why such patients are believed to have gynaecological disorders rather than an irritable bowel. My own work(7)on the reproduction of a patient's abdominal pain by balloon insufflation concentrated on perhaps the most enigmatic group of all - women with long-standing right upper quadrant pain. They shared many characteristics - fat intolerance and intolerance to a range of other foods, flatulence and dyspepsia. Most had been thoroughly investigated and many had already been given treatment for a range of disorders none of which, in the final analysis had proved relevant to their symptoms. Some patients had been found to have gallstones for example, but cholelithiasis had not produced lasting pain relief. 22 consecutive patients attending the gastroenterology department complaining of long-standing right hypochondrial pain were included in the study. They were mostly women and in the middle years of life with pain that had been present for many years, either intermittently or continuously and the radiation of pain was such that a biliary tract disorder would be suspected. These 22 patients shared an astounding total of 76 consultant referrals to either physicians or surgeons in the past and had been grossly over investigated. In total they had had 150 imaging investigations of their abdominal organs and 16 of the 22 had undergone 38 operations, all of which had proved unnecessary or unrelated to the patient's complaint. There had been 10 cholecystectomies (only 5 of them for gall stones), 12 appendicectomies (only one appendix showed acute changes of inflammation) and various gynaecological procedures. Transient symptomatic relief was sometimes achieved but no long-term benefits. Using a balloon to distend the alimentary tract from the oesophagus through the small intestine and round the large intestine it was possible to reproduce these patients' spontaneous abdominal pain in all but one case, the commonest trigger zones being the small intestine and the right colon. Half the patients had more than one trigger zone, not necessarily in continuity. This implies that functional gut pain can be caused not just by colonic sensitivity but by sensitivity in other parts of the gastrointestinal tract too. Furthermore, if these patients had been closely questioned on previous occasions it would have been found that the majority of them had symptoms suggestive of a functional disorder (wind, bloating, irregular bowels, pain relief related to defaecation) . More importantly,there had been a failure to assess the psychological status of these patients. Using a modified Hamilton rating scale(8) , half of the patients in our study were either moderately or severely depressed, a diagnosis which had not been entertained at any time along the course of their disorder.

Careful analysis of symptoms in patients with right upper quadrant pain serves to dispel the still prevalent myth that symptoms such as flatulence, heartburn, fat intolerance and non-specific abdominal pain are pathognomic of gall stone pathology. Bainton(9) interviewed a thousand patients on the electoral roll at Barry about these symptoms. Following cholecystography he was able to show that not only are flatulence, heartburn, fat intolerance and abdominal pain common, but they were no more common in those with stones than in those without stones. This, of course, is not new. In fact studies like this have frequently been reported over the past 40 years, but have been largely ignored.(10) Bockus said in 1946 that dyspeptic symptoms occurring day after day are rarely due to cholelithiasis and Alvarez in 1943 (11) said that "such symptoms are usually due to functional disease of the gastrointestinal tract and are not connected with the gall bladder" .

Similar caveats can be applied to pain in the right lower quadrant. Ingram(12) recorded that only 40% of the appendices removed by his team over a four-year period showed any histological evidence of disease, a figure which had been consistently reported in all previous studies. The sample contained a preponderance of young women and further analysis showed that 50% of appendices removed from young women who had acute abdominal pain were abnormal compared with only 11% of pathological appendices removed from those undergoing elective operation for chronic abdominal pain.

Psychological assessment carried out by a lady almoner within a day or two of operation was correlated with the histological findings, and it was found that two-thirds of the girls with very few emotional problems had a diseased appendix, but of those who complained of many emotional problems in only 17% of cases was a diseased organ removed. The same issue had been addressed by Creed (13) from a slightly different perspective. He interviewed all young post-appendicectomy patients between the ages of 15and 30 in three local hospitals, then followed them up a year later. Of those deemed to have been depressed at the time of their operation and in whom the appendix that was removed was normal, 80% of them still had their abdominal pain a year later compared with 20% of those who were not depressed at the time of their operation and whose appendices had been inflamed. Gomez and Dally(14) psychiatrically assessed 96 consecutive patients from medical and surgical clinics with abdominal pain within a week of their original presentation. Only 15 of these patients had organic disease and the remainder were thought to have predominantly psychological causes of one sort or another underlying their pain. When reviewed one year later, the diagnosis was changed in only one patient. One carcinoma of the colon turned up in those 81 patients. The most frequent psychiatric diagnosis in both the Barts series (Libby) and that reported by Dally was depression. Rose et al(15) looked at a hundred consecutive patients attending a medical clinic, 44 of whom reported abdominal pain as their main symptom. 33 out of these 44 patients (75%) were suffering from depression as measured by the Beck depression inventory. This was a study done by gastroenterologists who were accustomed to diagnosing depression clinically but despite this they missed at least 50% of these diagnoses clinically.

Are surgeons as good at diagnosing depression as their colleagues in gastroenterology, neurology and psychiatry? It is difficult to find any data on which to base an assessment. The following pharmacy returns from the University Hospital of Wales in Cardiff over a period of eight months speak eloquently.(16)

Table 1. Prescription of psychotropics by non-psychiatrists.

	Total	General Surgeons	Gastroenterologists
Antidepressants	196	3 (1 .5%)	73 (37%)
Anxiolytics	93	2	5
	289	5 (1.7%)	78 (27%)

In view of the paucity of data on the surgical approach to psychological problems I will conclude with the views of some eminent past physicians.

Sir Clifford Allbutt in 1884 (17) railing against the "tyranny of the gynaecologist" warned "arraign the uterus and you fix in the woman the arrow of hypochondria, perhaps for life". Hutchison, a little later, in 1923, coined the rather apt expression "abdominal woman". He did not reserve his invective for gynaecologists but points the finger at physicians and surgeons as well "the road to chronic abdominalism is paved with operations". His prophetic, if somewhat cynical view of treatment was to "dislocate the patient's mind from its perpetual revolution around her umbilicus". But let's give the last word to a surgeon. Mr C Jennings Marshall (18), writing in the Lancet in 1935 on the chronic abdomen, says categorically that in his mind surgery has no place in the treatment of the disease. "I am aware that the stomach, liver, kidney and colon-stitchers, the appendicectomists and the adhesion-dividers still claim results. They well can, for there is almost always improvement for six months."

References:

1. Bloomfield AL, Polland WS. Experimental referred pain from the gastro-intestinal tract. Part 11. Stomach, duodenum and colon. *J.Clin Invest* 1931; 10: 13: 453-73.
2. Bentley FH Smithwick RH. Visceral pain produced by balloon distension of the jejunum. *Lancet* 1940; 2: 389-91.
3. Waller SL, Misiewicz JJ. Prognosis in the irritable bowel syndrome. *Lancet* 1969; 2: 753-5.
4. Libby G. - Personal Communication.
5. Swarbrick ET, Hegarty JE, Bat L, Williams CB, Dawson AM . Site of pain from the irritable bowel. *Lancet* 1980; 2: 443-6.
6. Whorwell PJ, McCallum M, Creed FH, Roberts CT. Non-colonic features of irritable bowel syndrome. *Gut* 1986; 27: 37-40.
7. Kingham JGC and Dawson AM. Origin of chronic right upper quadrant pain. *Gut* 1985 ; 26; 8; p 783-788.
8. Hamilton M.A rating scale for depression. *J Neurol Neurosurg Psychiet* 1960;23 :56-2.
9. Bainton D. Gallbladder disease. *N Engl J Med* 1976; 294: 1147-9.
10. Price WH. Gallbladder dyspepsia. *Br Med J* 1963; 2: 138-41.
11. Alvarez WC. (1943) Nervousness, *Indigestion and Pain*. p.49. Heinemann, London.
12. Ingram PW, Evans G, Oppenheim AN. Right iliac fossa pain in young women. *Br Med J* 1965; ii: 149-51.
13. Creed FH. Life Events and Appendicectomy. *Lancet* 1981; ii: 1381-85.
14. Gomez J, Dally P. Psychologically mediated abdominal pain in surgical and medical outpatient clinics. *Br Med J* 1977; 1: 1451-3.
15. Rose JDR, Troughton AH, Harvey JS,et al . Depression and functional bowel disorders in gastrointestinal outpatients. *Gut* 1986: 27; 1025-1028.
16. Rose J. Personal Communication.
17. Allbutt TC. Neuroses of the Viscera. *Br Med J* 1884: 1; 495-499. 595-49.
18. Jennings Marshall C, The Chronic Abdominal Invalid. *Lancet* 1935; 908-909.

Discussion

Audience: What role do you think high sphincter of Oddi pressure has in chronic right upper abdominal pain? Some data from the States shows that in some cases sphincterotomy lowers the pressure and relieves the pain.

Kingham : The data are interesting. Doubtless, if functional disorders do occur in the alimentary tract they can occur in any part where there is smooth muscle. Smooth muscle is only found in certain parts of the biliary tract - the sphincter is one and the gall bladder another. At the present time the data is inconclusive but it seems reasonable that some patients suffer from this.

Dawson : This is an idea which has been around for some time. French surgeons in the '50s did a lot of work in this area but the idea was dropped because it did not fulfil the promise that was hoped for. Perhaps it is now possible to define the subgroup of patients who will respond to sphincterotomy better.

Audience : Referring to the work with young female appendicectomy patients, were you not surprised that 20% of the non-depressed group who had inflamed appendices removed still reported abdominal symptoms a year later?

Kingham: Yes I was and, in fact, no comment was made about why that should have been.

de Dombal : Several surveys of negative laparotomy patients have shown a consistent 20% of patients with residual morbidity, so perhaps the operation itself is implicated. Although a relatively minor procedure, negative laparotomy is not without a certain morbidity. In each of these series between 30% fnd 50% of patients came back, not after the first two or three months but after much longer periods from six to thirty-six months.

Dawson : A colleague of mine interviewed a group of patients post-operatively to time the recurrence of pain and found that it varied from three weeks to eighteen years with a mean of eight months. It is extremel difficult therefore to decide what is a reasonable follow up period. A 20% estimate is close to the proportion of the general population with abdominal symptoms which Ken Heaton has found in his survey.

Kingham: Do you think that just as we recognise a post-dysenteric irritable bowel triggered by an inflammatory reaction, it is also possible to get a post-laparotomy functional bowel syndrome?

de Dombal: That is a distinct possibility but until a long term prospective study is set up we will not know the answer. A recent paper in the American literature gives even more cause for concern in that younger women who had had negative operations were later found to have a higher carcinoma risk. If that finding is substantiated surgeons should not merely be barred but should carry a government health warning!

Audience : Assuming operations produce remission of symptoms for around six months, what are the result of treatment with antidepressants? Can these patients be persuaded to take antidepressants?

Kingham : It is remarkably difficult sometimes to convince these patients that there is a psychological component to their disorder. One of the more positive things to come out of the balloon insufflation work was that by reproducing pain in this manner patients were more convinced about a functional explanation. I have no data on long term follow-up of psychiatric treatment but it has the advantage of being less invasive than surgery.

Libby : We have not yet published our results from St Bartholomew's hospital but we have ten year follow-up data on the group of people you referred to in your presentation and at least half of them are completely well both psychologically and somatically. In relation to the somatisation of affective states it is not necessary for the patient to accept the functional nature of their disorder for treatment to work. As long as treatment is initiated the patient does not even have to be told they have a disturbed affect.

PELVIC CONGESTION IN YOUNG WOMEN: HAVE WE FOUND THE ANSWER?

Professor R Beard
Professor of Obstetrics and Gynaecology
St Mary's Hospital, London.

If a woman complains of pelvic pain then, in my experience, there is nearly always a somatic cause for it. The fact that the cause is often elusive does not negate the existence of pain. As a gynaecologist with a long-standing interest in pelvic pain of unknown origin in young women, in the reproductive period from 15 to 50 years, I believe that it represents a very neat model for psychosomatic disease and affective disorder. A multidisciplinary approach is essential for research in this area. At St Mary's my team includes gynaecologists, psychologists, endocrinologists, counsellors and specialists in measurement techniques. Today's meeting, which brings together people of many different persuasions with a common interest in studying abdominal pain goes some way towards addressing the problem and perhaps we should consider establishing a society of abdominal pain to pool the resources of the various specialities, in an ongoing way.

Taylor (1), an eminent American gynaecologist, surmised that no problem in clinical gynaecology presents more difficulty than that of pelvic pain occurring in the absence of any perceptible pathology. A man with an enquiring mind, he recognised that failure to detect the source of the pain did not mean it did not exist. A survey of 21,000 cases undergoing laparoscopy (2) found that the major cause (52%) for the procedure was pelvic pain. In other studies only 25% of women laparoscoped exhibit pathology, not necessarily the cause of pain, and in 75% no obvious abnormality is detected, so it is not surprising that gynaecologists find this a difficult area to manage and often refer these patients on to their gastroenterological colleagues.

For many years the French have believed this to be a condition which is associated with congestion, a common finding at laparoscopy. This is usually dismissed by gynaecologists as being a normal phenomenon because it occurs as a result of pregnancies but, in fact, pelvic pain with no obvious cause occurs just as commonly in the nulliparous as in the parous woman. The large veins illustrated in the venogram in figure 1 are not a normal finding in women who have no pain. So we set about trying to characterise this apparent vascular abnormality.

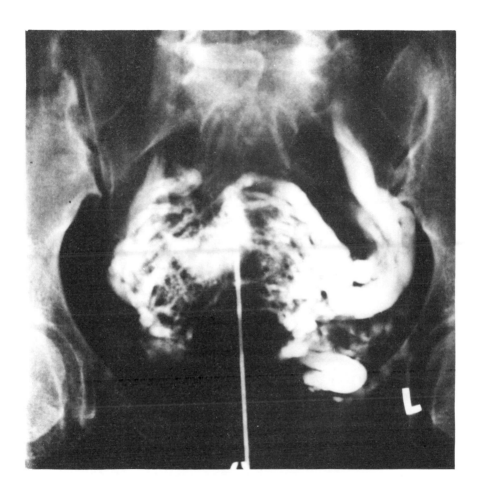

Figure 1. Venogram showing congestion in the left ovarian plexus.

The network of pelvic veins is a complex one with many functions to subserve ranging from orgasmic responses to sexual intercourse, to the very large volume of blood that they have to carry in pregnancy (a 70-fold increase in venous drainage) and the changes that occur during the menstrual cycle. In common with the venous drainage of the abdominal cavity, the pelvic veins have neither adventitial sheaths nor valves, essential features of a drainage system that has to respond to very large changes in blood volume. One of the techniques that we have used to look at this question is pelvic venography performed via a cannula introduced through the cervix up to the fundus of the uterus.Through this a needle is advanced into the myometrium and 20 ml of urograffin is injected over about 2 minutes.

In a normal woman nearly all the dye disappears very quickly after injection. Posture influences venous drainage to some extent but even in the erect position the dye is normally cleared within 20 seconds. The stage of the menstrual cycle also influences the state of the ovarian veins producing selective venodilatation of the ovarian vein on the side of the developing follicle, but this gradually returns to normal and the physiological dilatation that occurs is never of the magnitude commonly seen in women with pelvic congestion. Where pelvic congestion exists the picture is very different with large dilated veins on the periphery of the uterus, accumulation of dye bilaterally in the ovarian plexuses and slow clearance of dye indicating very marked stasis in the circulation of these women complaining of pelvic pain.

When women with unexplained pelvic pain were compared with both those in whom some pathology had been identified and a control group who had nothing wrong with them we showed a high degree of specificity (91%) and sensitivity (82%) for the venogram in selecting out women with pelvic congestion. (3) However, venography is an invasive technique so we now make more use of ultrasound scanning; for example, polycycstic ovaries are a very common finding (56%) in women with pelvic congestion, pointing to the central role of ovarian dysfunction in this particular problem.

Taylor (1) originally suggested that women with pelvic congestion have uterine hypertrophy - an observation that we have actually reproduced in a large series of women comparing a control group selected from the general population with those with pelvic congestion. The uterine size of those with pelvic congestion was 30% above the mean of the control group and this was excluding confounding variables such as the presence or absence of polycystic ovaries, and the parity of the woman. Generally speaking, regardless of whether these women have polycycstic ovaries or not, they have a bigger uterus than those in the control group.

Turning next to the symptomatology, it is important to emphasise that pelvic congestion and irritable bowel syndrome are two separate conditions although they can become confused and some women can be wrongly diagnosed. Pelvic congestion is quite clearly a condition associated with the reproductive period of life; (4) and that fits with our own findings that the ovary is the centre of the problem.

The classical presentation of pelvic congestion is pain, typically a dull ache interspersed with intermittent acute episodes, often resulting in women being admitted to hospital with suspected appendicitis, acute pelvic inflammatory disease or an ectopic pregnancy. The pain is often in the iliac fossa tending to occur only on one side, but careful enquiry will ellicit the history of occasional similar episodes on the other side. This differentiates the condition from endometriosis or appendicitis where the pain is usually reported only on one side. The pain is exacerbated by standing for long periods or walking. Using a vacuum cleaner seems to be a particularly uncomfortable activity. The pain is alleviated by lying down which fits in with descriptions by 19th century gynaecologists of these women being slaves to the chaise-longue .(5) They tend to be symptomatic also with backache, vaginal discharge and headache - 94% in our group had 2 or more symptoms, 69% reported congestive dysmenorrhoea, 50% had intercourse less than once a week, compared with only 15% of the control group and they commonly had deep dyspareunia. Most typically of all they often report postcoital ache, pain that comes on after intercourse, sometimes of great severity and maybe one of the factors which leads to the infrequency of intercourse. 60% of our sample suffered from chronic emotional disturbance. The most helpful physical sign is reproduction of the pain by pressure on the ovarian point which is located at the junction of the middle and upper third of a line drawn between the umbilicus and the anterior superior iliac spine. The pain is thus referred pain and this can be easily demonstrated during venography.
Pressure over the ovarian point diverts dye to the contralateral ovarian vein and reproduces the pain in the ovarian plexus by inducing back pressure. On speculum examination a very congested cervix is seen often with an erosion and an excess of white discharge due to excessive desquamation of vaginal epithelium. So in summary, the clinical findings are ovarian point tenderness in 77% of patients, movement of the cervix producing pain in 46% as compared with 6% in the control group, uterine tenderness in 57% as compared with 6%, and very typically, gentle pressure on the ovaries reproducing the pain that they have. Quite often this is the first time anyone has actually been able, at physical examination, to reproduce the pain. Given this combination of history and symptoms and signs, particularly postcoital ache, dysmenhorrhoea and ovarian point tenderness, you can very specifically diagnose pelvic congestion without turning to other investigations.

There is a strong relationship between emotional disturbance and the occurrence of pelvic congestion. Duncan & Taylor (6) showed that 29 of a group of 36 women had quite serious emotional deprivation in childhood - death of a parent before the patient was 12, separation or divorce of the patient, psychosis, alcoholism, serious parental discord, patient rejected by the family and chronic invalidism. A recent article (7) suggests that about of women presenting with this condition have a history of sexual abuse in childhood. In one of our own randomised control trials of the psychological aspects,(8) with up to six months follow-up we compared stress analysis and pain analysis, two different forms of therapy, against a control group who were simply reassured that there was no major disease. (Fig 2). Venograms showing congestion in several women have been shown to return almost to normal at follow-up a year later after psychotherapy, so psychotherapy does work but it is a time consuming activity and there is a need for an alternative solution.

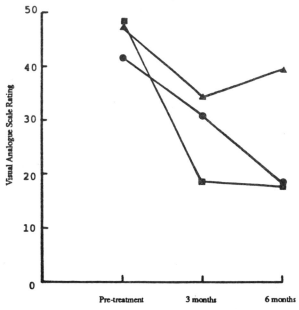

Figure 2. Visual analogue scale ratings of pain intensity pre-treatment, 3 months and 6 months after treatment commenced. Reproduced with permission from Pearce, 1986.

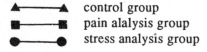

    ▲———▲ control group
    ■———■ pain alalysis group
    ●———● stress analysis group

So we turned to dihydroergotamine (DHE), which is a selective veno-constrictor, on the basis that if congestion is the cause of the problem, then by venoconstricting the veins in the pelvis, we might actually improve the condition. Reginald et al (9) reported the outcome of a group of women with pelvic congestion on venography who were given one milligram of DHE. All women showed a 30% diminution in the calibre of their pelvic veins with a consequent more rapid clearance of dye. If our hypothesis was right, then it would be logical to assume that these women would also experience some pain relief. We tested this hypothesis with a prospective trial in which women presenting with acute abdominal pains who were known to have pelvic congestion, were given either saline or DHE intravenously in a single blind manner then on the next occasion they presented with pain they were crossed over to the opposite treatment. Each time they were asked to score their pain response. The saline treated group showed a small placebo effect, but there was a much more marked immediate effect with DHE followed by persisting pain relief. We now use an oral form of DHE for treating women who present with postcoital ache and dyspareunia. Whilst useful in the short term for treating the acute condition in the long term the goal should be the suppression of ovarian function if indeed our hypothesis is true that ovarian dysfunction is the underlying problem. Medroxyprogesterone acetate was used in a pilot study and it produced about 80% suppression of ovarian function. We are currently completing a large randomised prospective trial of psychotherapy and medroxyprogesterone acetate. With adequate suppression of ovarian function pain scores for most women were reduced to a minimum. The problem with this form of treatment is that when treatment is withdrawn pain often returns over the next few months. What we are now finding is that if patients stay on the treatment until they themselves feel confident enough to stop and have a clear understanding of what causes the pain and how to manage it (usually after about a year on treatment) many of them are then able to come off the treatment and they have no further interference with their daily life.

Our hypothesis remains one of underlying ovarian dysfunction frequently associated with polycystic ovaries, dilated pelvic veins and an enlarged uterus, all of which lead to vascular congestion, pain and stress. Stress in turn affects the pituitary via the hypothalamic stimulation and leads to what I hypothesise to be an inappropriate secretion of LH with resulting ovarian dysfunction. Having very clearly demonstrated part of the equation, much endocrinological and careful psychological research remains to be done to elucidate the central mechanisms. When this is done we will have demonstrated a very nice model for psychosomatic disease, which underlines many of the conditions under discussion, including the irritable bowel syndrome.

Is there a place for surgery? In a small group of women we have had to resort to removing their ovaries and all 15 of them have been pain free to date. Two types of women present for surgery: those who have an intact uterus and ovaries in whom removing the ovaries with the uterus seems very beneficial, and a very large group of women who have had a hysterectomy with ovarian conservation in whom the ovaries are densely bound down to the side wall of the pelvis and the pain is certainly caused by the inability of ovulation to occur freely. They present with very large follicular cysts and are perhaps the women who respond best .They will tell you that this is the first time they have been free of pain for years. So there is a place for surgery, but only after medical treatment has failed.

References

1. Taylor H C. Vascular congestion and hyperemia II:The clinical aspects of congestive-fibrosis syndrome. *Am J Obstet Gynaecol* 1949; 57 : 637-653.
2. Chamberlain G, Brown J C, eds. Laproscopy. A report of the Working Party of the Confidential Enquiry into Gynaecological Laparoscopy(1978). Royal College of Obstet Gynecol,London.
3. Beard R W, Highman J H, Pearce S and Regionald PW. Diagnosis of pelvic varicosities in women with chronic pelvic pain. *Lancet* 1984; ii: 946-949.
4. Levitan Z, Eibschitz I, de Vries K, et al . The value of laparoscopy in women with chronic pelvic pain and a 'normal' pelvis. *Int J Obstet Gynaecol* 1985; 23: 71-74.
5. Gooch R (1831) *On Some of the Most Important Diseases Peculiar to Women.* pp 299-331. Republished by the Sydenham Society, London, 1859.
6. Duncan C H , Taylor H C A psychosomatic study of pelvic congestion. *Am J Obstet Gynecol* 1952: 1-12.
7. Harrap-Griffiths J, Katon W, Walker E, et al . The association between chronic pelvic pain, psychiatric diagnoses and childhood sexual abuse. *Obstet Gynecol* 1988; 71: 589-594.
8. Pearce S. (1986) *A Psychological Investigation of Chronic Pelvic Pain in Women.* Ph D Thesis. University of London.
9. Reginald P W, Beard R W, Kooner J S, Mathias C J, Samarage S U, Sutherland I A, and Wadsworth J. Intravenous dihydroergotamine to relieve pelvic congestion with pain in young women. *Lancet* 1987 ;*ii:* 351-353.

Discussion

Audience: A large number of irritable bowel patients have symptoms similar to your patients. Did any of your patients complain of bowel symptoms? Did you specifically ask about bowel symptoms?

Professor Beard: Very much so. There probably are a proportion of women in the irritable bowel group who actually have pelvic congestion and these should be identifiable using the techniques I have described. From our point of view, having investigated our group of women fully and localised their abnormality do they also have symptoms suggestive of irritable bowel? Surveys we have conducted since visiting Ken Heaton's unit and realising there could be some overlap suggest that the incidence of bowel and bladder symptoms is really rather low - in the order of 5%. Bloating is one interesting feature to have emerged.

Kingham: There are some aged observations in the literature on the effects of various forms of emotional stress on the vascularity of the gut, Beaumont's work on gastric fistulae for example, and the medical students' responses to being told they have colonic carcinoma half way through sigmoidoscopy. Changes occur, but they are not necessarily associated with any symptoms. Could it be that in the women in whom you have demonstrated pelvic congestion this is not necessarily responsible for their symptoms. It might be occurring pari passu the pain but not necessarily causing it.

Beard: The answer to your question revolves around another question - why are these veins becoming dilated? I believe that there is over-exposure of the ovarian veins to prostaglandin I2 which is a vasodilating hormone. The veins nearest the ovaries are most affected because of high local concentration of oestrogen. Further away from the ovaries the veins become less and less affected. Furthermore, although most of the drainage goes via the ovarian vein a proportion of venous blood travels via other vessels and may actually traverse the bowel drainage systems so it is not inconceivable that there might be a relationship between the two. This might account for the symptom of bloating which is the predominant bowel symptom reported in our surveys.

Moriarty: Another symptom akin to bloating is proptosis, a condition emphasised several years ago by Dr. Dawson. I wonder whether some of the women in your sample were suffering from proptosis with arching of the back and squeezing of the diaphragm producing distension.

Beard: Perhaps so but when you suppress ovarian function, they lose bloating.

CAN WE AUTOMATE THE DIAGNOSIS OF LOWER ABDOMINAL PAIN AND WHAT ARE THE PROBLEMS?

F T de Dombal
Reader in Clinical Information Sciences
University of Leeds

Automation has contributed to many areas of human endeavour so it is not unreasonable to suppose that it might have positive benefits for the complex area of medical diagnosis. The general public has a touching faith in the doctor's capacity for information processing which falls far short of reality. Automated decision-making aids, whilst quite unable to replace the doctor, have much to offer, both as educative systems for developing deductive decision-making skills, and as aids to more accurate diagnosis.

Misdiagnosed acute abdominal pain rapidly evolves into recurrent abdominal pain. 11% of all patients attending casualty departments who are discharged undiagnosed return within six months and clearly these patients constitute a major problem in that, although they present ostensibly with acute abdominal conditions, they actually suffer from a much more complex disorder. To make matters worse, many of these people undergo unpleasant and invasive investigations and even, in many cases, unnecessary operations. Procedures themselves carry a certain morbidity and operations may have long- term sequelae which are not immediately apparent.

Negative laparotomy rates in the U.K. as measured by various surveys can range as high as 60%. In Germany the negative laparotomy rate is of the same order but can go as high as 81% in young women. In fact, Litchner and Pflanz (1) demonstrated a correlation between negative laparotomy rates and mortality rates due to appendicitis and its treatment. 33,000 laparotomies are performed annually in the U.K. and, despite being considered by some to be a relatively minor and uncomplicated procedure, there are 100 deaths annually from negative laparotomies. In terms of resources this consumes about fifteen million pounds of National Health Service funds. Even more arresting is the suggestion from several sources that half of all deaths due to appendicectomy are preventable.

Our own efforts over the years have been focused on trying to improve diagnostic accuracy. The doctor collects information which he then feeds into a computer which analyses and displays various information and finally the doctor makes a decision with regard to assessment of symptoms. We found that junior doctors usually confine their enquiry even about obscure presentation of pain to 6 or 7 questions, some of which were of dubious

Abdominal Pain Chart

NAME		REG NUMBER	
MALE FEMALE AGE		FORM FILLED BY	
PRESENTATION (999, GP, etc)	DATE		TIME

PAIN

SITE		AGGRAVATING FACTORS	PROGRESS
		movement	better
ONSET		coughing	same
		respiration	worse
		food	DURATION
		other	
		none	
			TYPE
		RELIEVING FACTORS	intermittent
		lying still	steady
PRESENT		vomiting	colicky
		antacids	
		food	SEVERITY
		other	moderate
RADIATION		none	severe

HISTORY

NAUSEA	BOWELS	PREV SIMILAR PAIN
yes no	normal	yes no
	constipation	
VOMITING	diarrhoea	PREV ABDO SURGERY
yes no	blood	yes no
	mucus	
ANOREXIA		DRUGS FOR ABDO PAIN
yes no		yes no
	MICTURITION	
PREV INDIGESTION	normal	♀ LMP
yes no	frequency	
	dysuria	pregnant
	dark	
JAUNDICE	haematuria	Vag. discharge
yes no		dizzy faint

EXAMINATION

MOOD	TENDERNESS	INITIAL DIAGNOSIS & PLAN
normal		
distressed	REBOUND	
anxious	yes no	
SHOCKED	GUARDING	RESULTS
yes no	yes no	amylase
COLOUR	RIGIDITY	blood count (WBC)
normal	yes no	computer
pale		urine
flushed	MASS	X-ray
jaundiced	yes no	other
cyanosed		
TEMP PULSE	MURPHY'S	DIAG & PLAN AFTER INVEST
	+ve −ve	
BP		
	BOWEL SOUNDS	
ABDO MOVEMENT	normal absent	(time)
normal		
poor nil	RECTAL — VAGINAL TENDERNESS	DISCHARGE DIAGNOSIS
peristalsis	left	
	right	
SCAR	general	
yes no	mass	
DISTENSION	none	
yes no		

History and examination of other systems on separate case notes

Figure 1. Data collection form as used in the recent multi centre study to record data from patients with acute abdominal pain.

relevance. So the first task consisted of designing a form for data collection which was thorough, comprehensible and reproducible (Fig 1) .

The chaotic manner in which history taking often proceeds became apparent when we used 3 independent observers to record questions which were asked by doctors of patients with recurrent abdominal pain. 1 in 5 of all questions asked were phrased in such an ambiguous manner that the 3 observers were unable to reach consensus about what question had actually been asked. To confound matters further, 1 in 6 of the patients' responses were so vague that it was impossible to record a clear Yes or No answer. If we are to progress in our understanding of abdominal pain it is thus essential that a great deal of attention is paid to defining symptomatology and also to ensuring that young surgeons and physicians in training learn early how to elicit these symptoms. The computer's role is essentially to absorb this information and compare it with a bank of data stored in its memory in order to calculate a probability which is then displayed. A computer so programmed can distinguish between surgical abdominal pains, specific surgical disorders and non-specific abdominal pain.

Does this method of analysis actually pay dividends? A recent major survey (2) shows very clearly that it does. Diagnostic accuracy can be improved not only in the group of patients incorrectly diagnosed as having surgical pain, but also for those whose acute appendicitis was mistaken for non-specific recurrent pain (Table1) .

	Baseline (4075cases)	Trial Period (12662 cases)
Initial diagnostic accuracy	45.6%	65.0%
Post-investigation diagnostic accuracy	57.9%	74.2%
% NSAP* patients admitted from A/E**	40.9%	26.3%
%NSAP patients reattendedA/E	7.4%	1.5%
% NSAP patients operated on	9.5%	5.6%
Perf. appendicitis rate	23.7%	11.6%
Annual Saving Negative Laparotomies	-	139p.a.
NSAP bednights	-	3387p.a.
Appendicitis bednights	-	871p.a.
Bad Management errors	0.9%	0.2%
Death	1.20%	0.92%

*NSAP is Non Specific (Non-Surgical) Abdominal Pain, patients whose symptoms rapidly resolve and in whom no specific cause (and particularly no cause warranting surgery) is found.
** In the UK the Emergency Room is referred to as the " Accident & Emergency Department".

Table 1. Summary of findings in recent DHSS Trial of Computer-Aided Decision Support System for Acute Abdominal Pain.

Negative laparotomy rates decreased from 9.5% to 5.6% and the proportion of acute admissions for abdominal pain reduced from 40% to 25%. Mortality also decreased. The overall number of unnecessary operations can also be significantly reduced.

Diagnosis in children is more difficult,and young women pose problems in that gastroenterological disorders often become confused with gynaecological ones. However, by collecting appropriate information about gynaecological symptoms this distinction can also be made successfully by the computer, the differentiation between an ovarian cyst and acute appendicitis for example. So, the automated diagnosis of abdominal pain has been shown to reduce errors in the acute situation. But what about chronic conditions? One of the anomalies here is that as it becomes easier with time,to diagnose life-threatening and serious ailments such as cancer so the cure rate decreases! The ideal situation is one in which it would be possible to select at an earlier stage and with certainty the occasional serious pathology from the less serious gastroenterological symptoms presented by about 10% of the population. Some time ago we addressed this problem by selecting patients with gastroenterological symptoms from five Health Centres for closer follow-up. Patients with persisting complaints unresolved after two weeks of simple treatment were referred to a special clinic and underwent all the diagnostic procedures available. Out of the whole group 27 patients were found to have cancer of which 26 were correctly identified by the battery of tests. Diagnostic accuracy was certainly achieved but there was a prohibitively high false positive rate. It is a somewhat chastening experience therefore to discover that a nursing sister armed with a computer programme can achieve higher levels of diagnostic accuracy than specialists with all their diagnostic aids.(3) Her false positive rate was also high but not as high as with the battery of tests. Based on this experience the early targeting of suspicious patients becomes a distinct possibility. The penalty for extensive investigation rests not with the financial costs incurred but with the time for the patient. Macadam showed there was a median delay of 22-46 weeks in diagnosing gastroenterological cancers which is potentially avoidable if patients could be screened when they first present and only those with a high index of suspicion of cancer shunted immediately into high technology investigations (4).

How should the computer be used to present its results? Some advocate using the computer in the same way as a special diagnostic test. Others expect it to behave like a substitute specialist. The most appropriate role for automated diagnosis has yet to be defined. So have the problems. There are medico- legal problems, not least being the issue of system security. But the main problems relate to liability for use - who is to blame if the computer gets it wrong - and liability for non-use. If a doctor chooses not to use a system which improves diagnostic accuracy is he then more liable for his errors?

From an educational point of view, it is interesting to consider briefly why a doctor's diagnostic skill should improve when he uses an automated aid. A 10% improvement in relatively inexperienced junior staff is commonly observed in a short period of time with the computer and is an eloquent argument in favour of their use. It is achieved quite simply by imposing a high degree of discipline on the process of data collection and a standardised framework for interview and examination. The repercussions are twofold - in their educational impact and in their stimulus to good practice. Textbooks and teaching that emphasise the classical presentations of advanced disease are not only inappropriate, but counterproductive. There seems little use in being able to diagnose with certainty a cancer that has progressed to the stage where intervention is impossible and palliation the only option. What we should be doing is replacing these dated descriptions with descriptions of early stages of disease and how to recognise them. The British Society of Gastroenterology has just spent 5 years collating data and delineating the clinical features of a very large series of patients with early gastric cancer. The educational contribution of automated data collection is immense.

Finally, the most useful aspect of all has little to do with automation but a lot to do with good clinical practice. It stems from experienced physicians and surgeons making their collective wisdom accessible to those who are relatively inexperienced. We have nothing to fear from numbers, and a sensible attitude to decision-making aids can only be of benefit, especially in an area such as recurrent abdominal pain where complex interdisciplinary diagnostic problems are involved. Automation is not a substitute for our own judgement but a way of combining our talents, not so that we end up talking to computers but so that we are better able to talk amongst ourselves.

References.

1.Litchner S, Pflanz N. Appendectomy in the Federal Republic of Germany: Epidemiology medical care patterns. *Med Care* 1971, 3:911.

2.Adams ID, Chan M, Clifford P.C. et al. computer-aided diagnosis of acute abdominal pain: a multi-centre study. *Brit Med J,* 1986; 293:800

3.Clamp SE Wenham JS. Interviewing by paramedics with computer analysis: Gastrointestinal Cancer. In:Rozen P, de Dombel F T, Karger S, eds. *Frontiers of Gastrointestinal Research. Computer Aids in Gastroenterology.* , Basel, Switzerland 1984;110-118.

4.MacAdam DB. A study in general practice of the symptoms and delay patterns in the diagnosis of gastrointestinal cancer. J Roy *Coll of Gen Pract* 1979 ; 29:723.

DISCUSSION

Beard:I agree that the education component is actually one of the most important aspects of computerisation because it trains junior staff to ask a whole range of questions routinely. Why don't surgeons use the laparoscope?

de Dombal:I suspect it is because they do not consider gynaecology. (There has been a flurry of correspondence in the BMJ recently about people with vascular problems presenting with bellyache. The diagnostic accuracy for such cases is about 20% mainly because the doctor never thinks the patient may have a vascular problem.) If you want to ensure a negative laparotomy, the best way to do it is to take a young woman who's got a gynaecological problem and send her to the surgical ward. The gynaecological aspects are overlooked - because of compartmentalised thinking.

Beard: The point is though that when it comes to appendicitis you can very beautifully see the appendix through the laparoscope with no problem at all.

de Dombal: In acute abdominal pain a reasonable modus operandi for an inexperienced doctor would be to take a decent history, make a proper physical examination (using techniques approved and agreed in advance by a consensus of his peers) and thereby triage patients into 3 groups: those with an obvious acute abdomen; those who obviously have little the matter with them and then a group in the middle. That is the group who would benefit from laparoscopy.

Moriarty: This approach could also be extended to the primary care situation. There was a very good study, (1) published last year by three GPs in Salford who looked at 150 patients with abdominal pain, including children, of whom 9 were referred as emergencies. Of these 9, 8 were admitted to hospital and all were referred to surgeons rather than to gastroenterologists. In the final analysis, only 3 patients had a surgical condition. So it is not just the junior doctor in A & E who needs guidelines, GPs could benefit as well.

de Dombal: As you rightly say, theirs is a difficult and different problem. A GP once said to me, "It's alright discharging patients from hospital and saying they're not surgical. Your problem's finished, mine's just started." There was a very interesting paper looking at life events and stress and depression scales in controls and patients with and without appendicitis reported in last month's Gut. We have actually done some work along these lines giving HAD scales to patients with and without appendicitis and found, much to our surprise, there didn't seem to be much difference between the two groups.

Audience: Your work obviously has great relevance for medical audit. It is easy in many instances to say when a surgeon has not performed well, be it a negative laparotomy or he might kill a patient. It's not nearly so obvious when a physician practices badly, for example, ordering an inappropriate ERCP. Does your work have any application for calling physicians to account?

de Dombal: I doubt if anybody here in this room can actually define good medical care. The thing that worries me about an audit is not that it is designed to promote good medical care (whatever that might be) but that it is imposed on us from outside the profession - and we have thrust upon us performance indicators, some of which are totally irrelevant to the actual clinical care of the patients concerned.

Your question is, however, crucial, because I think what we have to do in every area of clinical medicine is to define clearly undesirable events. This is what we've done for surgery. If you are dealing with the situation, for example, where somebody presents with acute abdominal pain, then (1) you don't want them to die, (2) you do not want them to have an operation if they haven't got appendicitis, (3) you don't want an 8-hour delay if they do have acute appendicitis and (4) you want them out of hospital in 10 days with no complications. It's much more difficult to apply to the care the physician gives - which is why we need to get together and form multidisciplinary groups to examine these problems. I feel very strongly that if we don't do this and report back maybe through the colleges and actually take the initiative we shall have audits thrust upon us from outside.

Feinman: My particular interest is chronic pain and if you compare patients with trigeminal neuralgia with patients with atypical facial pain on the HAD scales, those with trigeminal neuralgia have much more depression and anxiety than the patients with atypical facial pain. This reinforces your point about the complexity of medical care. All pain is distressing but the emotional disturbance which is produced is more complicated than depression or anxiety per se.

Heaton: That is a very important point. The simple fact of having chronic, unrelieved pain may itself induce depression, and we shouldn't too readily blame our patients' pain and other symptoms on depression when, as so often occurs, they have done the rounds of doctors and specialists who have been unable to give them a diagnosis. Earlier in the day someone expressed the view that we might be missing the wood for the trees and that instead of worrying about what happens in the abdomen we should concentrate on what is happening in the head -that it's all in the mind. In fact, if you survey the general population although you find a high proportion of people with IBS symptoms, only 20% of them have been to see a doctor. The great majority are not anxious or depressed, at least, not enough to go and see a doctor .(2) Two excellent American studies have just been published which have looked in great detail at the psychological profiles of non- reporters of irritable bowel syndromes by comparison with the general population and have found no difference .(3,4) Everyone accepts that the reporters, the cases we see in our clinics, are very often depressed, but there are other possible reasons for that as I have just mentioned. But the non-reporters are psychologically normal. Furthermore, IBS can develop in situations which have nothing to do with psychology - the post-dysenteric variety of IBS, for example, and the post-cholecystectomy IBS and some IBS which is simply caused by constipation. So, I think we must be very careful about putting it all up in the mind.

Beard: The American Surgeon General some years ago commented on the age discrepancy between appendicectomies in men and women. The operation was commoner in women, and there was an enormously increased prevalence between the ages of about 16 and 24 amongst the girls which almost certainly relates to the new experience of menstrual function, dysmenorrhoea and ovulation. It raises interesting questions about why some and not all girls present with acute abdominal pain, and I think this compartmentalisation between psychological factors and somatic ones is what we need to break down because the two are clearly interrelated. I'd like to put forward the hypothesis that some people are more sensitive to stress, they react more strongly to a standard stress or pain stimulus, that is, they complain more about it. The women who consult us about pelvic pain have a higher incidence of depression and are more neurotic when they have the pain than at other times which begs the question - is it the pain that's causing it, or is it the influence of the childhood factors we alluded to? I think it's a combination of both, but what seems to happen is that when they are cured and they are pain free, they score relatively normally on the psychological scales.

Dawson: The effect of depression on pain perception is quite marked. Everybody agrees that depressed people perceive pain differently and it maybe very difficult to distinguish between the cart and horse.

Beard: Depression in this group comes from the fact that they've met barriers to progress in the management of their problem, and when you do solve it, you clear that.

Dawson:I'm not sure that this is always so, because very often when taking histories of patients with recurrent abdominal pain you'll find mild affective swings going on a year or two before the pain starts, and if that is so, one can't say the depression is reactive to pain. Obviously some are reacting to pain as in carcinoma of the pancreas, the classic example of organic gut disease mistreated as depression. Before the advent of the imaging era a laparotomy was occasionally considered appropriate for someone with depression and recent onset abdominal pain.

Beard: Certainly the life events studies would support that.

Libbey: You're both right. You can have a depression and you can also be frustrated by lack of proper care. You can have irritable bowel and depression or any combination of circumstances.

Audience: As far as pain perception in IBS patients is concerned has it not been shown that during cold immerson IBS patients were more resistant to pain than normal controls?

Kingham: There was a paper in Gastroenterology within the last few months (5) showing that they didn't have decreased pain tolerance. This was not confined to depressive irritable bowels, it was just irritable bowels without particular psychological overlay.

Moriarty: The cutaneous pain threshold of patients with irritable bowel syndrome was in fact higher than that of normals. The same was also true of patients with Crohn's disease.

Heaton: Pain was induced in this study by passing electric current through the hand, and it has been pointed out that thresholds for visceral pain may be different from cutaneous pain.

Dawson: The work on differences between visceral and cutaneous pain was carried out in the 30's by Chester Jones and his Colleagues.

Wingate: In the first series of IBS patients we studied at the London-Hospital we did psychometric testing to see how disturbed they were psychologically. And to our surprise when compared with a control group of patients from the gastroenterology clinic with benign organic diagnoses such as reflux oesophagitis and healthy controls we could find no difference in any parameters, except perhaps anxiety because they were uncertain about what was wrong with them. I believe our approach was very important, in that we were investigating then on the assumption that they had a detectable motility disorder and there was no suggestion of depression or psychological disturbance. Many of the studies reflect the frustrations patients feel when they meet doctors who are equally frustrated by their patients, in other words the psychometric indices simply reflect a flawed doctor-patient relationship .

Moriarty: Some clarification of the terminology may help to dismiss some peoples' reservations about using psychiatric labels in the diagnosis. We recognise organic pain, we recognise factitious pain, such as the patient with Munchausen's syndrome, but what people object to is the label "functional pain" or "irritable bowel". Part of the reason for this is that traditionally the word "functional"has been used interchangeably with the word factitious to imply that the pain is made up or that the pain is in the patient's mind. Describing the irritable bowel syndrome as a "functional gastrointestinal disorder" implies that there may be an underlying pathophysiological process. But the irritable bowel is not a disease, it is a syndrome, and such a large proportion of the population have it, that it deserves to be considered as part of the range of normality. Professor Wingate's experience is at variance with that of most of the published studies, which have reported that patients who present with IBS do exhibit health care seeking behaviour and did rate highly on anxiety and depression scales.

Heaton: But what exactly is the mechanism of the symptoms? I absolutely agree that this is essentially a syndrome, a collection of symptoms but nevertheless, there is evidence to show that there is a pathophysiological abnormality. There is work which suggests the existence of gut hyperreactivity similar to the hyperreactivity of the bronchi in asthma for example. It's certainly been shown in the rectum and no doubt Professor Wingate will enlarge on this area later, but if that is true, then despite the frequency of the condition in the general population, we must accept that there is something abnormal pathophysiologically, and that it's not simply an increased awareness of normal events.

Kingham: That goes slightly against your own findings. In your Bristol study where 30% of local factory workers have these symptoms it is nonsense to define that as abnormal if only 60% of the population are not having them.

Heaton: The true figure for IBS, the classical IBS, in terms of recurrent abdominal pain relieved by defaecation is nearer to 13%.

References

1. Edwards MW, Foreman WM, Walton J. Audit of abdominal pain in general practice. *J R Coll Gen Pract* 1985; 35:235-8.

2. Thompson WG, Heaton KW. Functional bowel disorders in apparently healthy people. *Gastroenterol* 1980; 79:283-8.

3. Drossman DA, McKee DC, Sandler RS, et al. Pyschological factors in irritable bowel syndrome: a multivariate study (Abstract). *Gastroenterol* 1987; 92 (5 pt 2): 1374.

4. Whitehead WE, Bosmajian L, Zanderman A, et al. Role of psychological symptoms in irritable bowel syndrome: comparison of community and clinic samples (Abstract). *Gastroenterol* 1987; 92 (5 pt 2): 1693.

5. Cook IJ, van Eeden A, Collins SM. Patients with irritable bowel syndrome have greater pain tolerance than normal subjects. *Gastroenterol* 1987; 93:4:727-33.

PHYSIOLOGICAL ASPECT OF RECURRENT ABDOMINAL PAIN

D L Wingate
Professor of Gastrointiestinal Science
The London Hospital Medical College

Until recently little was known about the physiology and neurophysiology of the gut. The classical model for studying the gut dates from the nineteenth century concepts of Beaumont, Bernard, Bayliss and Starling for whom the gut was an inert tube responding only when stimulated. Basal parameters would be measured -secretion, motility absorption or whatever was being evaluated - then the stimulus, usually a meal, was applied and the change in activity measured. The gastroenterology and pharmacology journals are still publishing experiments of this design which presuppose the gut is an inert organ responding in a simplified way to stimulation.

Boldyreff, in 1902, working for his PhD thesis under Pavlov, studied pancreatic secretion in much the same way as Bayliss and Starling except that he observed the basal period for much longer and discovered that this was not a period of inactivity, but that the stomach underwent episodic bursts of contractions every 90 minutes until interrupted by food when the pattern changed to repeated regular contractions.

This was evidence of at least two different states of activity in the stomach only one of which was dependent on the presence of food. After arousing initial interest, this aspect of gut motility was largely ignored until, in the 1960's, the technique of studying conscious animals using electrodes implanted in the wall of the gut was pioneered at the Mayo Clinic. Joseph Szurszewski, a neuropharmacologist, published the landmark paper (1) reporting repetitive bursts of EMG activity recurring at 90 minute intervals throughout the gut and migrating distally. These coincided exactly with the phenomenon described earlier by Boldyreff.

The next piece of the jigsaw was provided by a distinguished American physiologist, Dr Charles Code, who published a paper in 1975 reporting the effects of food on the system. When dogs were fed the change in the pattern of motility occurred simultaneously throughout the gut. He also drew attention to another type of activity preceding the regular burst of contractions in which the gut contracted irregularly during a period of relative quiescence. The periodic repetition of three phases of motor activity - quiescence, irregular contractions and regular contractions - appearing to migrate from stomach to ileocaecal sphincter is now known as the migrating motor complex (MMC). The motor activity of the gut is organised as migrating motor complexes in nearly every mammalian species so far studied.

Carnivores

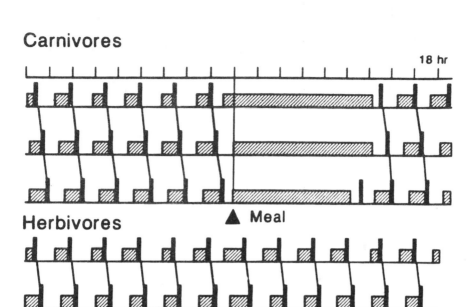

Herbivores

▲ Meal

▲   ▲ ▲   ▲   ▲ ▲   ▲   Fodder

Figure 1
Schematic representation of MMC sequence at 3 levels of the small bowel in (above) carnivores and (below) herbivores. Black triangles indicate timing of feeds. Each MMC icon consists of a shaded portion representing irregular activity (Phase 2) followed by a vertical bar indicating the brief phase of regular contractions (Phase 3); the space between successive icons is the p phase of motor quiescence (Phase 1). Note that in carnivores, but not herbivores, feeding induces a prolonged period of (Phase 2-like) irregular contractions.

Carnivores with their once - daily, highly concentrated nutrient load needing chemical digestion vary in pattern from herbivores who continuously graze on a high bulk, low nutrient diet (Fig 1). For them propulsion plays a larger role. So the MMC seems to be the main pattern of organisation of motor activity of the bowel which serves to propel material along the gut and is, for example, important for emptying solids larger than 1mm from the human stomach. A different kind of pattern is required for complex chemical meals which are low in bulk and high in nutrient value. My own interest in the field developed in response to this new aspect of physiology - a control system whose dysfunction might account for the symptoms reported by patients with recurrent abdominal pain.

Hypotheses about gut hormones abounded in the mid 1970's but it is now clear that the control system for gut motility lies not with hormones but with a highly specialised branch of the autonomic nervous system called the enteric nervous system (ENS). Langley originally proposed the ENS as a division of the autonomic system along with the sympathetic and parasympathetic divisions but it was, until recently, largely ignored. Traditional teaching described gut control in terms of sympathetic inhibition and parasympathetic stimulation. Meissner's plexus and Auerbach's plexus received little attention but we now know that these constitute the enteric nervous system. The myenteric plexus, lying between the longitudinal and circular muscle layers is perhaps the most important and reaches from the distal portion of the oesophagus to the dentate line of the anus. The submucosal plexus is the second most important network. These plexuses consist of ganglia with interconnecting fibres and cell bodies - an extremely unusual arrangement for a peripheral nervous system. Moreover, ENS innervation is dense; estimates range from 5 to 100 million neurons, certainly as many as are found in the spinal cord, but arranged in this characteristic way, seen elsewhere only in the cerebral cortex.

Within the enteric system there are both adrenergic and cholinergic fibres but the majority of the putative neurotransmitters are amines such as 5H-T or serotonin, substance P and VIP. Dynorphin, enkephalin, somatostatin, and CCK-octapeptide have also been identified but in smaller proportions. Many neurons contain more than one neurotransmitter or neuromodulator in specific combinations. Thus there appears to be some form of chemical coding involved. It is an extremely complex system in which different morphological types of neurones and chemically distinct neurones have different functions because they project in different ways.

In other words this is the "gut brain" . In terms of neuroanatomy and neurophysiology it has sensory neurones, motor neurones, interneurones and glia; glial cells are found elsewhere only in the CNS. It has a dense synaptic neuropil, multiple synaptic mechanisms including post-synaptic potentials, multiple neurotransmitter substances, a lack of connective tissue, little extracellular space and even its own blood brain barrier.

In functional terms it behaves in a complex integrative way like the "big" brain. There are sensory nerves and effectors - the enteric neurones provide all the smooth muscle innervation and certain stereotyped programmes of activity are set in motion by specific stimuli. Three such programmes have been well characterised so far. The first is the interdigestive or MMC programme which occurs when there is no food. The second programme is activated by the presence of food and the third stereotyped response, familiar to surgeons, is adynamic ileus in which quiescence occurs when the gut is handled and persists long after the stimulus has ceased. Ileus does not occur in patients with visceral aganglionosis.

However the enteric nervous system does not operate in isolation. Much of the sensory information from the gut by- passes the enteric nervous system to pass directly to the brainstem via the vagus nerve. 90% of the vagal fibres are afferent and only 10% are efferent, carrying information back to the enteric system. There are approximately 5,000 efferent vagal fibres supplying a population of 5×10^6 enteric neurons; clearly the influence of the CNS on the enteric system is limited and hierarchical with specific responses programmed peripherally rather than centrally. It does however point the way to understanding the connection between stress and gut reactions. If stress is conceptualised as abnormal perturbation of the CNS it is quite easy to see how messages from higher centres can modulate enteric programmes of activity. The two nervous systems are, in effect, wired together.

We have developed a technology for recording gut motor activity in conscious ambulant patients over lengthy periods of time. A fine nasojejunal tube is passed which is attached to a small portable recording instrument which can easily be carried about the person without interfering with their daily routine. Recordings made in this way clearly demonstrate the effects of CNS arousal on the gut nervous system. Phase 3 activity slows down at night and the irregular phase 2 type of activity disappears altogether during sleep. This indicates a diurnal rhythm in vagal tone present during the day but absent during sleep. In normal people, psychological stress interferes with the enteric nervous system as shown by the fact that MMCs are substantially diminished during a couple of hours of acute mental stress only to reappear immediately the stressful stimulus is removed .(2) We then studied small bowel motility of patients with IBS (3) , since it is not yet possible to study the colon in this way. We detected a rhythm of clustered contractions in IBS patients, but not in controls, with clusters of 3 or 4 contractions every minute for up to 2 hours. When these occur in normal subjects they rarely persist for more than 5 or 6 minutes at a time. These prolonged clusters were seen in 18 out of 22 patients in our first series, usually during controlled mental stress, and then in 11 out of 12 in a second series of IBS patients. This deviation from the normal MMC pattern only occurs in the waking state and is often accompanied by pain.

The value of the ambulatory technique is that we are able to study patients for several days at a time in their own environment, subjected to their normal stresses and strains. In a laboratory or clinic bed they are often symptom-free for the 6 hours of the study.

So, what does all this have to do with pain? Quite possibly what is happening during the periods of disordered motility is that small segmental obstructions develop with pain due to distension and raised intraluminal pressure. Thus, if I were to speculate on the mechanism of pain production in IBS, I would say the source lies not in the head but in the gut. It derives from disordered motility in people who are more vulnerable to stress and is probably the result of a mildly damaged enteric nervous system - for example, in those with post-dysentery IBS - the CNS thereby more easily causing disruption. Life, for the gut, is a struggle between the "little brain" and the "big brain" and sometimes the battle can be very painful.

References

1. Szurszewski J H. A migratory electrical complex of the canine small intestine. *Am J Physiol* 1969; 217: 1757- 1763

2. Valori R M, Kumar D, Wingate D L. Effects of different types of stress and of 'prokinetic' drugs on the control of the fasting motor complex in humans. *Gastroenterol* 1986; 90: 1890-1900

3. Kumar D, Wingate D L. The irritable bowel syndrome: a paroxysmal motor disorder. *Lancet* 1985; ii: 973-977

Discussion

Kingham: When did the patient start complaining of pain on awakening, was it immediately or was there a delay? How do you know the pain was not continuing during sleep?

Wingate: If pain is a sensation, and you are unconscious I am not certain whether it's possible to suffer pain while you're asleep. What we know is that this disturbance of the normal programme of motor activity does not occur during sleep in IBS patients. When it does occur during sleep, it is in people who have severe enteric nerve damage, which is how we now diagnose enteric neuropathy.

Beard: I'm not quite sure why you assign a primary role to neurological damage. Firstly, in a condition that occurs so commonly in the population, it seems most unlikely that there is underlying pathology, and secondly, is there any objective histological evidence of damage?

Wingate: When you see abnormal patterns in a system like this it has to be associated with nerves because gut smooth muscle can only contract when commanded by a nerve. By definition then this is a neural dysfunction. It is extremely difficult to determine whether this is due to actual nerve damage. We need a method of taking full thickness biopsies in people who are not ill enough to need surgery. Until we are able to look in detail at these plexuses with silver staining we will not know the answer. With regard to your comment about prevalence I believe this arises out of diagnostic confusion about irritable bowel syndrome. If you lump all unexplained abdominal dysfunction together and call it irritable bowel syndrome unless it's gynaecological, then irritable bowel syndrome is very common. If you define it a bit more carefully, exclude people with dyspepsia-type syndromes, and concentrate on people who have erratic defaecation and associated abdominal pain, the numbers actually get rather smaller.

Audience: What happens to the clusters of activity with feeding? In herbivores, is the pattern innate?

Wingate: The pattern is clearly related to diet. If you take a pig, which is an omnivore, and you feed it fodder, it behaves like cows, and if you give it a Big Mac and French fries, it behaves like man. But the clusters of activity I described are seen only in IBS patients at the end of the post-prandial period and during a fast.

Audience: What is the influence of the limbic system on the nucleus of the vagus nerve as a part of the CNS integration of information.

Wingate: That's a big question to answer. The nuclei of the vagal nerve are in the brainstem but the influence of the limbic system is exerted via the efferent arm of

41

the vagus nerve. We know that integration occurs at the level of the limbic system. Neurophysiologically, other levels of integration have been demonstrated in the hypothalamus and brain stem where there is convergence of signals from different gut receptors.

Moriarty: Just to put the enteric nervous system into perspective, it has become clear to me through my work on the neurohumoral regulation of intestinal fluid transport that the dominant influence is still the parasympathetic with its modulation from the sympathetic. Not by chance are both the cranial and sacral parasympathetic fibres involved. Cerebral events are likely to be very important and it is a mistake to concentrate only on the gut. These abnormalities that you describe in the colon in irritable bowel syndrome have also been described in patients with no symptoms of irritable bowel syndrome, but who have a comparable degree of psychoneurotic traits. This implies that the motor abnormality in the colon is a reflection of psychological disturbance or depression, rather than being a physiological abnormality associated with the irritable bowel.

Wingate: It isn't true to say that there is a characteristic change in the colon that's been described in irritable bowel syndrome. If it had been we would all know what we are talking about. There have been patterns described in the colon in IBS that have also been found in normals and in psychoneurotics, but there is no colonic motor pattern pathognomonic of IBS. That is one of the problems. We do not even know how to record from the colon. The data that we've shown here in IBS patients has been replicated at the Mayo Clinic using pharmacologic challenge by injecting neostigmine and CCK in IBS patients.

Moriarty: What about this dominance of the parasympathetic over the role of the enteric? How important is it in motility? The enteric system contributes relativey little to the regulation of intestinal fluid transport.

Wingate: If you autotransplant a piece of gut which is completely isolated from any nervous influence at all it will still show migrating complex activity. So, it must be the enteric system which drives motility. But it is modulated by the CNS, because the periodicity is different after transplant. The programmes are inherent; that same piece of gut will also go into ileus.

Audience: The physiology seems to be born out in practice. We see very few of our irritable bowel patients who are woken at night by pain, whereas, for example, a peptic ulcer patient does wake up. I'm not sure I understand the cause of the pain in that either. Have you done any studies in patients with peptic ulcers?

Wingate: Using technology that was not as good, we could find no relation between pain and motility nor was the motility in ulcer patients in any way different from those of normal controls.

42

PSYCHOGENIC FACTORS - AETIOLOGY AND MANAGEMENT

J P Cobb
Consultant Psychiatrist and Senior Lecturer
Institute of Psychiatry London

Introduction

Over the past 2 years I have had the opportunity to assess and treat 16 patients with irritable bowel symptoms. The link between psychiatric problems and an irritable bowel is widely recognised and for some patients their disorder remains intractable and persistent. They tend to be referred to numerous specialists including gastroenterologists, general physicians, endocrinologists and particularly gynaecologists before they reach the psychiatrist if they ever do. By this time they have undergone frequent investigations and their abdomens are criss-crossed with laparotomy scars. Macdonald and Bouchier (1) reported that 40% of their patients with notable psychiatric illness (8 out of a series of 19 patients) still had problems at 12 months follow-up. In a classic paper by Chaudhary and Truelove (2) in which they excluded those with dysentery from their group of irritable bowel patients and concentrated on those with psychiatric symptoms, only 26% were better at the end of the follow-up period. So not only is this an enigmatic condition, it is also a persistent one.

Aetiology

Structural Aspects

Certain personality characteristics occur frequently in IBS patients. Beard (3) showed that pelvic pain patients scored higher on the neurotic scale of the Eysenck Personality Inventory. Several authors, including Macdonald and Bouchier (1) observe that those with obsessional personalities are particularly likely to develop these problems.

Psychiatric Illness

A proportion of IBS patients have associated psychiatric illness, most commonly but not exclusively, depression and anxiety.

Intra-personal Difficulties

Beard (3) referred to patients who had negative views of themselves and people with chronic abdominal pain tend to have poor self-esteem, to be unassertive and to have difficulties with sexual relationships.

Interpersonal Difficulties

Chaudhary and Truelove observed that many patients with irritable bowel had experienced a situational change - most commonly a change of job or a divorce - and on the whole these people did well.(2)   Creed and ∠ennard-Jones (4) analysing patients who had had negative appendicectomies, noted a high rate of family difficulties and recent interpersonal stress.

Treatment

Little has been written about the treatment of functional abdominal pain. A brief paragraph in Hill's book (5) on psychosomatic disorders discusses the value of a supportive and understanding physician in the long-term management of these patients. Creed (4) talks more specifically about accepting the reality of their symptoms.

If a patient is told "there is nothing wrong with you", then their perplexity and anxiety is often increased. Despite the absence of organic pathology

PSYCHIATRIC DIAGNOSIS	COBB	MACDONALD (1980) and BOUCHER	GOMEZ(1977) and DALLY
	n=16	n=28	n=96
HYPOCHONDRIACAL ANXIETY	2	11	21
GENERALISED ANXIETY AND PANIC DISORDER	2		
DEPRESSION	3	14	31
FUNCTIONAL PAIN (HYSTERICAL)	1	1	17
RELATIONSHIP PROBLEMS	4	-	-
INTRA-PERSONAL PROBLEMS	4	-	-
NIGHTMARES	1	-	-
BULIMIA NERVOSA	2	-	-
FEAR OF SOILING	1	-	-
OBSESSIONAL PERSONALITY	6	-	-
ALCOHOL	-	1	12
BEREAVEMENT	-	1	-
SUBSEQUENT ORGANIC DISORDER	-	-	15

Table 1. Comparison of psychiatric diagnoses between three series of patients.

the psychic experience of pain is real enough. Creed also emphasises the importance of explaining mechanisms.(4) Reassurance is best avoided but ways of helping the patient to develop self-reassurance are encouraged. Relaxation and desensitisation are particularly useful for those patients who experience clearly defined, episodic discomfort related to particular situations.

Patient population
Of the 16 patients who have been referred to me over the past 2 years with functional abdominal pain there were twice as many women as men (F=10, M=6) and they were mainly young people aged between 23 and 52 years (average 35 years) . 13 of the group had a medical diagnosis of IBS, 1 had gastritis, 1 had reflux vomiting and 1 had constipation. Most of them had suffered from their condition for long periods of time ranging from 1 - 20 years with an average of around 9 years. They were a chronically disabled group of patients.

In terms of psychiatric diagnosis these patients were typical compared with those reported by Macdonald and Bouchier (1) and Gomez and Dally (6) as Table 1 shows. Only four of my 16 patients reported a significant degree of anxiety. Two of these were hypochondriacal anxiety related to their abdominal pain and the other two reported anxiety symptoms but did not see any relationship between their anxiety and their gut symptoms. Depression too was much less common in my group. The high incidence in functional pain reported in Gomez and Dally's group is at variance with the experience of others and is therefore questionable. Relationship problems and intra-personal problems were present in a significant proportion of my patients, perhaps reflecting my own particular bias. Nevertheless, I think it would be true to say these problems are only identified if they are specifically looked for, they do not occur more frequently than previously reported.

Nightmares were directly related to IBS in one patient who experienced pain during the nightmare which would then awaken him to bowel symptoms. The nightmares involved pursuit and torture, being stabbed, and once, being conveyed across the atlantic on the nose of a 747 which crashed because of his weight. He recognised that these dreams reflected his tendency to brood and see himself as vulnerable and would probably have responded well to therapy had he stayed.

Two patients had classical bulimia nervosa. One of them had actually been into hospital without revealing his symptoms to the investigating physician. His daily draughts of 200 mls Kaolin and Morphine for 2 or 3 days followed by ingestion of 12 bars of Ex-lax chocolate for the next 5 days had quite escaped notice. When he was in a purgative phase he would live on Coca Cola and Kit Kat biscuits whereas during a constipating phase he would eat anything and everything. Somehow he had managed to avoid mentioning any of this behaviour until his psychiatric referral. People are often reluctant to declare what they perceive to be shameful personal weaknesses. Another patient, originally diagnosed as IBS, was in fact afraid of soiling herself. She carried with her at all times a map of London with all the public lavatories in the areas she frequented clearly marked so she would never be far from a public convenience and this was clearly her main problem. Obsessional personalities were also overrepresented in this group and although I saw no alcoholics there is no doubt they exist in groups of IBS sufferers.

Methods of management

1 . Behavioural

Symptom rationale
Relaxation
Autogenic training
Cue analysis and modification
Training in coping skills/exposure
Bowel training
 Abreaction

2. Cognitive

Identification of automatic thoughts
Focus on underlying beliefs and attitudes
Challenging through empirical testing
Generation of alternative thoughts/beliefs

3. General psychotherapeutic methods

Identification of "inner conflicts"
Attention to interpersonal relationships
Problem-solving skills
Life structure

 4. Pharmacological treatment

Tricyclics: imipramine amitriptyline;lofepramine
MAOI: tranylcypromine+trifluoperazine (Parstelin);
phenelzine
Benzodiazepine: clonazepam

My own approach to treatment is an eclectic one. Two patients did very well with relaxation, another did well with autogenic training and one lady derived no benefit from either - hardly a surprising outcome considering her symptoms related to an unhappy marriage. Her husband, who had suffered a heart attack five years before, had been neglecting his business and spending time with a mistress. A dramatic exacerbation of her symptoms occurred when she discovered within a short space of time both the mistress and the deterioration of the business. But because, as she put it, "you cannot get angry with a man who has had a coronary", she had been unable to ventilate her anger for two or three years. What finally worked for her was a good therapeutic divorce.

Cue analysis and modification is a way of getting the patient to look at what precipitates their symptoms, and as part of engaging these patients I would usually invite them to keep a diary of symptoms including details of when the symptoms occur and what happens just before the symptoms occur to see if there are any recognisable precipitating events which in turn might lead to ways of modifying the symptoms.

Training in coping skills or bowel retraining can be illustrated by the patient who commented that the more she strained on the toilet, the more anxious she became and the more she feared incomplete evacuation. The approach in this case was to stop her from straining and to encourage her to sit on the toilet, perhaps reading a newspaper, smoking a cigarette, or having a cup of tea, but not actually trying to open her bowels. The instruction was paradoxical in that she was asked not to try to defecate at all.

Simple behavioural methods such as exposure can be effective in teaching alternative ways of handling distress or pain rather than taking codeine, which was quite popular among these patients. The lady with the phobia was persuaded to spend longer and longer intervals away from lavatories, and to eventually go out without a map. Other methods such as abreaction are more complex. One patient who had had a very traumatic childhood was unable to say the word, "mother." Whenever he tried to say it, he stuttered, so therapy consisted of making him repeat the word "mother" over and over again. When that occurred he in fact went into an intense emotional abreaction.

I also use positive methods, most commonly the elucidation and modification of underlying thoughts. One such thought is, "If I don't empty my bowel, I'll have a terrible day." Another common one is, "Well, even though the doctor's done all the tests there must be something wrong, maybe I have a tumour. "

Focusing on underlying beliefs and attitudes was the approach taken with an interesting girl, who was convinced, because of childhood experiences, that she would be a clumsy and ineffective mother and therefore should not get pregnant although at another level she very much wanted to conceive. She had suffered gynaecological problems for four or five years and also sexual difficulties. Her thoughts and beliefs were then challenged using cognitive approaches through empirical testing. Cognitive therapists describe themselves as collaborative empiricists which refers to their technique of working with the patient to set up certain experiments or tasks and then collecting data to see whether the thoughts and attitudes are valid or not. The next step is to generate alternative thoughts and beliefs.

There are some more general psychotherapeutic methods such as the identification of inner conflicts and relationship conflicts which are not always simple or direct. For example, one lady noticed that when her husband was away on business for a week or two she was free of symptoms, and when he came back the symptoms returned. The obvious (and erroneous) implication from this sequence was that there was something wrong with the marriage. In actual fact she had a very possessive, powerful mother, who totally disapproved of her husband, and the real problem centred on her guilt and her conflict about her mother, and her mother's relationship to the husband. When I saw husband and wife together they actually got on very well with each other. So the work began with changing her attitude towards her mother rather than focusing on the marriage.

Problem-solving skills can be effectively taught to those patients who are unassertive and unable to say no. They frequently dither obsessionally about decisions so one of the approaches here is to help them to be more assertive and to reorganise their lives in a more sensible way and to tackle problems in a constructive manner. In those patients with depression I use Tricyclics - either imipramine or amitriptyline if anxiety is prominent, although, unfortunately, the anticholinergic side-effects can sometimes aggravate the patient's symptoms. Of the more modern antidepressants, lofepramine seems to have least side effects. Parstelin also seems to be useful in this sort of patient as does phenelzine. As for the benzodiazepines, the only one I tend to use is the very long acting clonazepam which has a half-life of 24 hours. It is recommended for use in temporal lobe epilepsy, but is also proving to be of use in panic attacks and anxiety. Patients do still become dependent but it's much less of a problem than with either diazepam or lorazepam.

Outcome

Therapy time was usually 4 hours which included a one and a half hour assessment interview which in itself contributes to therapy. So overall therapy was relatively time economic considering that two of the patients in the 'definitely improved' group had had symptoms for 15 years. Before drawing definitive conclusions further follow-up will be necessary.

Symptom free	4
Definite improvement	5
Slight improvement	2
No change	2
Unknown	3
Worse	0

Table 2: Outcome of 16 patients after treatment course (approx 4 hours) at one year follow up.

Summary

Patients with functional abdominal pain are a fascinating and much neglected group. They are a heterogeneous psychiatric group including those with personality problems, with classical psychiatric diagnoses and with intrapsychic and interpersonal problems. Treatment, if it is to take account of this range, must be flexible, varied, and selected either according to clinical judgement or patient preference. Patients seem to respond to relatively short interventions and if improvement is going to occur it will do so within 4 or 5 hours of therapy. Of those who do not improve a few become long-term treatment problems. However, a long history of the condition does not necessarily infer a poor prognosis which is fortunate as psychiatric intervention often comes late rather than early if it comes at all.

References

1. Macdonald A J, Bouchier I A D . Non-organic Gastrointestinal Illness: A Medical and Psychiatric Study. *Br J Psychiatry* 1980; 136: 276-83.

2. Chaudhary N A, Truelove S C. The Irritable Colon Syndrome: A Study of the Clinical Features, Predisposing Causes and Prognosis in 130 cases. *Q J Med* 1962; 31:307-22.

3. Beard R W, Besley E M , Lieberman B A, Wilkinson J C M. Pelvic Pain in Women. *Am J Obstet Gynaecol* 1977; 128: 566-70.4.

4. Creed F, Lennard Jones J E. Gastrointestinal Symptoms. In: Medicine of Psychiatry - A Practical Approach. Pitman Books, 1981: 319-335.

5. Hill O W. Functional Vomiting, Abdominal Pain and Diarrhoea. Modern Trends in Psychosomatic Medicine. In: Hill O W, ed. Butterworth 1970: 147-63.

6. Gomez J, Dally P. Psychologically Mediated Abdominal Pain in Surgical and Medical Outpatient Clinics. *Br Med J* 1977; 1: 1451-3.

DISCUSSION

Dawson: What Dr Cobb has been talking about are the recidivists - a highly selected group who have not responded to explanation, reassurance and optimal dosage of antidepressants, which many do without being referred to a psychiatrist. So it's the hard core group of patients that one would not expect to get better at all who were the focus rather than the general unselected group of IBS patients.

Wingate: I find that a simple explanation based on the material I presented earlier is quite easy to get over to patients and it seems to help. More specifically it helps to eliminate the fear of cancer and you can sometimes be a great success even when a disorder has been long-standing. On the other hand, we have recently seen three patients who presented with classical features of IBS and all were shown to have quite severe gut disturbance with an underlying sensory neuropathy. Another, self-referred patient turned out to have severe motor disturbance manifested as nocturnal abdominal pain, so I don't think referral for psychotherapy would have helped any of these people. What is needed is accurate diagnosis.

Cobb: What interests me is the extent to which the disability experienced is out of all proportion to the underlying psychological or structural abnormality. Very often the patients I see do have physical abnormalities but the way they cope with them is unsatisfactory.

Wingate: I also find life events analyses of IBS patients generally unimpressive, but one of the things that does seem to occur frequently is threat from some future event which may actually never happen - a divorce, a child leaving home, retirement from a job. Often when patients return feeling much better and you ask whether the event occurred they say it happened and they got over it or else it never happened at all
.

Libby: As a psychiatrist who has actually been dealing with these patients for at least 10 years I do not think we should ignore the word "hysteria". The evidence from this symposium has shown overwhelmingly that depression is always occurring in these patients, be it from questionnaires, anecdotes, or whatever. Depression is disturbed affect, affect is feeling. Affect is the life blood, or the juice, if you like, of hysteria. Hysteria is a copying mechanism by which the human being deals with intolerable situations. If we expect to measure affect by questionnaires or sitting in the clinic talking to psychia ists, we'll certainly pick up some cases, but we are actually missing the point because the disorder with which they present - the pain - is actually there. Don't argue with the patient any more, it's there. Having accepted that premiss, the trick and the delight is in the treatment. In my experience these patients do not do as badly as Dr Cobb would have us believe. If you take the affective disturbance on board then that affect is movable. My approach is firstly to accept the disturbed affect then secondly to use any therapeutic manoeuvre - tricylic antidepressants, ECT, suggestion even cognitive therapy - to help the distressed person to shift his affect away from where it's presenting, which in these cases is in the enteric nervous system.

Feinmann: As a psychiatrist who has studied pain in a more controlled way I agree with Dr Cobb that these patients can be helped in a short length of time. What concerns me is that we, as psychiatrists, have become the surrogate history takers for other specialists and I don't see that as our role any more. It's about time other specialists started taking proper histories and finding out what has gone wrong with their patients in much the same way as Professor Beard does. By the time a patient with a psychosomatic symptom has reached a psychiatrist they've gone through so many consultations and investigations that it is very difficult to help them, whereas if they had been properly interviewed much earlier, we could prevent them from becoming chronic pain sufferers

Audience: There's a lot more to history taking than just asking a series of questions such as those in the Maudsley booklet. It is one of the most skilled things that psychiatrists do and not all interviewing can be delegated to nurses or computers or questionnaires. It may be appropriate to delegate the ordinary bread and butter of history taking but it's the interactive elements, getting people to talk about things that they find extremely uncomfortable, or embarrassing or painful, or things that they're only partly aware of themselves that are crucial.

Dawson: One of the problems is the lack of emphasis on studying psychosomatic disorders in training programmes for surgeons and physicians. It is just as important for a gastroenterologist to consider. Except for a few isolated members of each sub-speciality there is very little interest in this aspect of disease which is why patients get to the stage where they need to be referred on.

Cobb: You often have to overcome hostility. When I ask people what they think about coming to see me they often say, "not much", because they didn't want to come. There is often strong denial of a psychological problem.

Feinmann: They normally start with "I don't need a psychiatrist and I won't take pills."

Beard: Part of our problem in this educational issue is the conditioning of the 19th century, which basically said at last we have found what the cause of disease is - it's organic. And to get the population back to accepting that they've got some form of psychological problem is going to be a very difficult one, because it's now perceived as a weakness and something you don't admit to. I happen to agree with you that it is important to pay people to do these things, but it's not possible to do everything. I find that my time and my ability to do the psychological counselling is very limited and that's why we have counsellors who work in the clinic. That in itself is very important in that they should be seen to be an integrated part of treatment and patients will then feel much more secure about it. I have no doubt that counselling, good history taking, and therapy of the sort we try to provide is essential but it's very difficult to persuade the administrators who have to pay for counsellors of the value of this approach. We still have a long way to go.

de Dombal: Two issues have been raised which I wish to comment on. First, there are the people attending clinics who have not had a proper history taken. I suspect that there are an awful lot more people who do not have a proper history taken and do not get as far as your specialised clinic. These are the people who are truly dissatisfied with the care that they are given, because they don't actually have an opportunity to ever get it right. Secondly, this issue of funding is a very important one. Doctors' time is extremely valuable but if it takes an hour and a half to get a good history, we're not going to have the facilities to do it. What I'd like to suggest is that what we've seen this morning demonstrates to some extent that there are two levels of history taking. One is what we call the grammar of history taking, that is to say, making sure one simply asks questions by rote, doesn't miss anything obvious, doesn't miss the sensible questions. Then there is the prose of history taking, which is best left to the experts, the psychiatrists. It is probably not a skill which can be taught anyway.

Audience: There is not enough time in a normal working gynaecological clinic to elicit the information you're talking about. As a nurse with a health visiting background working in a gynaecological clinic I see the patients with problems that a doctor has recognised and referred on to me. I too spend an hour and a half with the patient and they often divulge a lot of relevant details. We then have access to a psychologist, which is also proving very positive. So it's not only money which is important but also time.

Wingate: It is so important to talk to patients. Quite often it is all that is necessary - I quite often don't examine the patients and very rarely do I do sigmoidoscopy in IBS patients. If you insist on doing investigations on patients that you know are going to be negative before you do them, there is definitely something wrong with you.

Audience:I refer patients to psychiatric colleagues when my own skills run out, which is not infrequent, but resentment can be a big problem. One of the best ways to avoid hostility, right from start when a patient walks into the room,is to introduce the idea that you're interested in his problems, before you even talk about the symptoms. What causes the biggest problem is when you investigate the symptoms and come to the end and say, well, we can't find anything wrong, now we'll have a look at the psychiatric aspects.

Libby: In my enthusiasm,I think I might have insulted Dr Cobb by implying that behaviour therapy or psychotherapy was not indicated. What I wanted to remind everyone was that the big brain itself gets upset from dysfunction, and that is called depression; very common, eminently treatable, and if you miss it, then psychotherapy and counselling and social work and understanding are all irrelevant and inappropriate.

Audience: No mention has been made so far of hypnotherapy, and there are some good comparative studies showing that hypnotherapy is superior to psychotherapy for IBS. What is the place of hypnotherapy?

Cobb: Relaxation, autogenic training and hypnosis all produce physiologically the same effect, and very often from the point of view of suggestibility, the deeply relaxed patient, or the patient doing autogenic training will be highly suggestible so they all seem to be points along a spectrum. In a way it is just semantics, so that inducing any state in which the patient is in a low state of arousal and suggestible can be a powerful form of treatment.

PRACTICAL ASPECTS OF MANAGEMENT

All speakers

Moriarty: An important issue which should be addressed is how far to investigate a patient. If you carry out a lot of negative investigations on patients it only serves to reinforce their fear of organic disease. A confident diagnosis should be made as early as is reasonably possible. I agree with Dr Dawson that a sigmoidoscopy in these patients is essential. If a competent clinician thinks the diagnosis is irritable bowel syndrome, then a normal full blood count and ESR and a normal sigmoidoscopy are all that are needed to ensure the diagnosis is correct 99% of the time. It behoves every physician seeing patients with abdominal pain to be able to take a short psychiatric history. This can be done quite effectively with a few simple questions in a couple of minutes

Cobb: If you are going to do that you might think of computerising it because you could possibly run those questions quite quickly in the waiting room and identify a certain proportion of patients with problems.

Moriarty: And perhaps as a screening tool which could be used quite effectively in out-patients.

de Dombal: We are setting about doing just that but there is no substitute for the intuitive feel a fully trained and skilled individual has. It does ensure however that simple questions are not overlooked.

Beard:I am interested to hear Dr Cobb, as a psychiatrist, suggest using a computer. The sort of questions that we have to ask about sexual dysfunction, sexual abuse and emotional deprivation in childhood are quite unsuitable for computerisation. I agree that we all need to take a short psychiatric history, but even that will not ellicit some of the essential information which our counsellors come up with and I don't think there are any short cuts to that.

Cobb: What I was reacting to was the appalling idea of a 2-minute psychiatric interview.

Moriarty: No, that is not what I meant. Given a patient with abdominal pain one has to use the first consultation time optimally and I would hope you can assess whether someone is normal within 2 minutes.

Cobb: Psychological assessment is a fairly long and skilled business, and it does need a lot of patience. We have an eighteen month full-time training course for nurses, and they need all of that.

de Dombal: This is right. One of the saddest things that came out of the-Glasgow computer experiments was the fact that when patients were interviewed afterwards the computer was perceived to be more sympathetic, more caring, and more worried about the patient's problem than the physician who interviewed them. We have actually come across the same phenomenon in our own experiments where we have asked our patients for a critique of the computer programme they have have used and the overall feeling is "thank goodness somebody cares about my symptoms". And I hate to take issue with anybody on the business of the 2 minute psychiatric interview but it seems to me that what is at stake is not the difference between a 2 minute psychiatric interview and a proper one, but between the 2 minute psychiatric interview and absolutely nothing at all which is what is happening at the moment.

Heaton: There's another element to that, too: the computer interview is a relevant interview. It questions patients about the things which are bothering them. It is a sad reflection on the quality of the average doctor's history-taking skills that many of the questions he asks are not relevant to the patient and their problem, and it's because of the mechanical way that medical students are taught, that they never quite get over going through a mechanical list of questions. To me this is one of the most important aspects of the skilled history taker that they can really focus on the complaint and analyse it and dissect it, and very often this is all that is necessary for the patient to feel that they have been taken seriously.

Wingate: Unfortunately the way medical students are taught reflects the way that the doctors who teach them think. Undue emphasis is laid on "objective knowledge" because it is easy to test by MCQ and examination. Medical students and the doctors who teach them share the delusion that this is somehow very important. The whole approach is wrong, it reflects on the teachers, it reflects on the teaching method and the examination system, and ultimately it reflects on the medical students.

Audience: The simple question, "What goes through your mind at the time you're getting symptoms?" often ellicits useful information and if you then go on to ask, "What do you think the symptoms are the result of?" you often get further relevant associations.

Audience: You don't necessarily need a computer facility. For the last 14 years every patient of mind has been given a self-administered health questionnaire to fill in. This means that at the time of the interview I don't have to ask all the standard questions - do they smoke, what did their granny die of, what tablets have they had - all that information has already been collected, and you can spend the time that they are with you concentrating on their problem. They've done all the clerking themselves. There's a complaints page on the front and some of them just write "bellyache", whereas others write two foolscap pages - but you can actually spend your 20 minutes with the patient looking at the psychiatric aspects or looking specifically at their bellyache and the rest is at your fingertips. It is filed in the notes and available for reference 15 years later. So you don't actually need a computer, just 6 pages of questionnaire.

de Dombal: We've tried both ways and I would accept that the importance is in the questions, not in the technology. I teach medical students by saying that if that's all you're going to do, I can get a device to do it at the speed of light. But don't you want to do more?

Audience: There are two very interesting questions on my list. One asks "Do you consider yourself to be unduly nervous or anxious" - to which 90% of all patients reply that they do consider themselves to be unduly nervous or anxious. And the other one asks "Are you depressed or not depressed?" and about 70% consider themselves to be depressed.

Audience:I'd like to ask the speakers whether they feel Colofac has any role in the management of irritable bowel, or whether it's a substitute for a good attitude and a good relationship with the patient?

Wingate: Any placebo about which both the doctor and the patient share a (maybe) deluded belief that it's going to work, is a very powerful placebo indeed. Colofac has a very high placebo effectiveness, because there are few alternative preparations available. It doesn't seem to be toxic or produce nasty side effects and there are very few specific therapies designed for IBS. It's been marketed as something specifically intended for the irritable bowel syndrome, but there's no reason why it should work. Why should a drug work on something whose pathophysiology is completely unknown? A decision was made that it works, this was accepted by the medical profession and communicated to the patients in a condition in which the placebo responses are very high, and Colofac elicits a very high placebo response. I certainly use it when I think that it will help.

Audience: Do you think that it is the Colofac or because you are a very nice person?

Wingate:I think it is the placebo effect. I think these things do help.

Beard: The problem with that is that many patients are not convinced by it. If you haven't revealed many details about the disorder but you assure the patient it's going to be good because we know it works, you get limited mileage on that. We spend a fair bit of time taking patients off Colofac and then investigating them.

Wingate:I would never give it to a patient and say, this is definitely going to help you. It may help them whilst they are undergoing further investigations,

Cobb: You can give your patients a diary and say, look, we are going to work out, you and I, whether this stuff helps. Start taking it. Then they become interested in their own problem, and in the management of their own problem. I think keeping a diary and looking at the way the symptoms fluctuate, is something that they go along with if you're giving them a questionnaire or using a computer for an interview or whatever.

Dawson: I don't think I've ever seen anybody who hasn't been given Colofac!

Libby: The key question is "How do you feel?" That is a challenge, because either they say they feel all right which belies the existence of their irritable bowels and suggests there may be a masked problem or they say they do not feel well in which case you have something to deal with.

Dawson:I quite agree. You can pick up a lot of information by asking "what's your general health like? How are you generally?" The patient then says, "Oh, I 'm not quite so good, " and you're away. In the ordinary general out-patient clinic that's one of the most important question to ask.

Moriarty:I think it's very important for us to drawn a distinction between the ordinary irritable bowel syndrome and those with intractable disorders, and it is possible to identify them with a few simple questions. If you ask people, are they happy, are there any sleep disturbances, is their concentration impaired, and enquire about emotional lability, and you get negative answers, then it's unlikely that you're going to miss serious psychopathology. Some years ago Ritchie and Truelove (1) did a trial of triple therapy in a group of patients with irritable bowel syndrome who were unselected in terms of underlying depression. All patients were treated with a fibre preparation, an antispasmodic and an antidepressant, and 70 to 80% of the patients responded well. It was one of the most efficacious courses of treatment ever given despite the non selective nature of the patients and a lack of emphasis on the psychopathology or the physiology.

Beard: In fact, when we did our fibre trial, we got the same results in the placebo group as we did when we gave the fibre. Up to 70% improved, and the trouble is this is a very suggestible group of people. Can I raise the question that possibly we are missing a small and important group. As doctors we assume patients come to us to get rid of their pain, but in fact, there is a group of people who need their pain. This was illustrated by a woman who came to see me with her husband, who was extremely attentive. She gave a history of having had an affair with a man whom she loved deeply but relinquished in order to make a success of her marriage. She needed her pain because it explained to her husband why she had gone from being young, attractive and well-dressed into a rather dowdy individual, who was depressed. The danger of taking away that pain was that she hadn't anything to fall back on, and I wonder what the psychiatrists have to say about how we should manage that.

Cobb: Well, this is obviously an interpersonal problem you would treat together with her husband, I suspect. It may be that she either has to choose between the pain or divorce.

Wingate: We can waste a lot of time trying to treat people who don't want to be treated so perhaps it is appropriate always to ask if they want to be treated and if so what kind of treatment they have in mind. One must not assume that a patient's only reason for consulting you is to get rid of pain. Sometimes they are simply looking for an explanation or an assurance. It is an important point.

Cobb: This is particularly true of the hypochondriacal anxiety group who are less concerned about the symptom than the fear of what it might be.

Audience: One of the questions I find helpful in understanding the patient is to ask myself "what purpose does this pain serve?" It is more acceptable often for a patient to cope with a physical or medical complaint than to discuss the real issue which may be incest or sexual abuse for example. The question is therefore an important one not just for counsellors, like myself, but for medical specialists working with pain.

Cobb: It has to be carefully put because it can sound quite perjorative. I tend to say, "What are the disadvantages of the pain?" and then perhaps move on to "could it be that the pain has any advantages?

Audience: Another way might be to ask, "How might your life or your relationship with your husband be different were the pain to stop tomorrow?"

Audience: Professor Wingate's view about the limitation of investigations prompts me to comment on the situation in the pelvic pain clinic at St. Mary's Hospital. At one time the drop-out rate for patients referred for psychotherapy was 40-50%. Since we started doing pelvic venography and the patient can actually see dilated vessels the current psychotherapy drop out rate is down to less than 20%, presumably because the pathophysiology has been demonstrated.

Wingate: Let there be no misunderstanding about what I said, which was: do not waste time doing investigations that you know will prove negative. What you are describing is a diagnostic investigation and is enormously valuable.

Heaton: Can I suggest there is something in common between the pelvic venography that Philip Reginald does and the motility studies that David Wingate does: both of them give the doctor confidence in handling the patient. And that, I suspect, has something to do with your better take up rate of psychotherapy, because you are more confident in your approach to the patient and in the way you present the information to them about what you think is wrong and what you think ought to be done about it. Being confident in the diagnosis is a fundamental part of managing IBS and that is why I put so much stress on the virtues of positive history taking, which enables you to make the diagnosis, with confidence, even without a diagnostic test. Dr Salter and others have done follow-up studies on IBS showing that it is a safe diagnosis, that you hardly ever miss organic disease.(2)

Beard: I think we are all agreed about the place of investigation but nonetheless I still have a big problem convincing patients that IBS is a safe diagnosis, although it can make them faint, and that it doesn't necessarily mean there is something seriously organically wrong. If we all had pelvic venography or the technology to show them a migrating electrical complex or what Dr Dawson described as sigmoidoscopy insufflation which reproduces the pain these would be very helpful. But we don't, so it is very hard to convince patients that recurrent pain doesn't necessarily mean that there's something terribly wrong. They have a perpetual fear that, because the pain is continuing, there must be something potentially serious causing it.

Wingate: Let me stress that we don't do sophisticated tests on all patients and nor is it necessary. The sort of heuristic model that I described is a conceptual model to explain to patients that there is a defect and that it may be a continuing defect, and therefore that may explain in itself why it goes on. I have the (perhaps mistaken) confidence of a physician who thinks he knows what the actual problem is, and in many ways that helps!

Beard:I think we do too! The question of age is absolutely fundamental and whilst we're all talking about functional disorders being so common it is important to emphasise that we are talking specifically about young people.

Wingate: Yes, that's right. The 50-year old patient who comes with a 3 month history of problems with defecation is an entirely different proposition.

Beard: But we still have general practitioners making a diagnosis of irritable bowel when the diagnosis is rectal carcinoma so your point about not examining the patient is slightly worrying.

Wingate: It's a selective policy.

Audience: In view of the neurobiochemistry you have described in the enteric nervous system are you aware of the development of any drugs which might be used in the same way psychotropics are used in the 'brain' ?

Wingate: One is dealing with similar neuronal networks and therefore it is conceivable that psychotropic drugs, which are effective at the CNS level will be developed which will be effective at the ENS level, and this may involve an ability to get through blood brain barriers or gut-brain blood barriers. However, the history of pharmacotherapy of neural dysfunction is not tremendously encouraging. Apart from the dopamine story the - probability of finding an effective drug which repairs a specific biochemical defect is not terrifically high. One has got to keep an open mind, but the successful drug will probably be a psychotropic. We know that the benzodiazepines, for example, are ineffective.

Beard: The only way forward in irritable bowel syndrome is to postulate that certain chemical agents, perhaps the prostaglandins, are implicated and a logical way forward would be to investigate these using selective anti-prostaglandins. It is rather sad that you dismiss that approach, because it seems to me it's one of the few approaches that you have in the human that is ethically acceptable.

Wingate: Well, I was asked to speculate. I wouldn't dismiss it, but if you ask me what I'm going to put my money on, I'm not going to put my money on that.

Audience: Listening to the discussion it sounds as if the gastroenterology clinic is going to be a sorting-out clinic for psychiatric patients. What does the panel feel about labelling patients as mentally ill? To a lot of people that still carries an unpleasant stigma.

Wingate: Yes. I've never dared refer an IBS patient to a psychiatrist. I don't think our psychiatrists would accept them. They'd say "Don't be so stupid, we've got serious work to do. " The stigma in the East End of London that is attached to seeing a psychiatrist is very considerable. That doesn't mean to say we don't recognise that a degree of psychiatric dysfunction exists.

de Dombal: Just to add a tangential, and only marginally abrasive note to this, I should like to agree with what you say. I've always regarded the prime function of a clinic to be the identification of serious diseases which require immediate attention, and only secondarily to deal with the group of patients we've been talking about today. We have deliberately excluded talking today about a whole range of patients who have cancer, who have peptic ulcer, who have inflammatory bowel disease, who have diverticular disease, which gives the false impression that the main concern of the clinic is to single out patients with functional disorders and to refer them to psychiatrists. We have been talking about a special sub-set of patients, and I do hope we have not given the impression that when one sits in the gastroenterology clinic and a patient comes in, the first thing that goes through ones mind is, "Should this patient go to the psychiatrist or not?"

Audience: Each patient thinks that his symptoms are more important than anybody else's in the world and while that patient is in the room with you, you have to concentrate on them alone, not on the next patient who might have cancer of the stomach or cancer of the pancreas (which you can do less about than the irritable bowel, incidentally). You have got to get that patient's symptoms better, that's what he came for. And I think you have all been somewhat dismissive of antispasmodics. We don't understand the pathophysiology of headaches but we still give aspirin for it, and we know it cures it.With a lot of these patients, if you use doses of antispasmodics that are sufficient, and usually the manufacturers recommendations are far too low, you can actually make the patients feel symptomatically a lot better, although you have no idea what the irritable bowel is.

References

1. Holmes KM, Salter RH. Irritable bowel syndrome - a safe diagnosis? *Br Med J* 1982; 285: 1533-34.

2. Richie JA, Truelove SC. Comparison of various treatments for irritable bowel syndrome. *Br Med* J 1980; 281: 1317-19.

List of Delegates - The Problem of Recurrent Abdominal Pain

ALSTEAD E M
London
ARCHBOLD J A A
Downpatrick
ARVIND A S
London
BASS C
London
BOWN R
Frimley
BRECKOR N
London
CAMERON D
London
CARMICHAEL H
Alexandria
CATNACH S
London
CHIPATO
London
CROWLEY S
London
FARQUHAR C
London
FEINMANN C
London
FORGE J
Enfield
FOWLIE S
Oxford
GANNON K
London
GEORGE N V
Rugby
GOETING N
Duphar
GOLDSMITH P
Barnet
HIMA
Maidstone

HINGIORANI K
Gateshead
HUGHES S
Winchester
JUSTINS D
London
KERRIGAN G N W
Newmarket
KING R A
Barnet
KIROLLOS W S
Kings Lynn
LECOYTE T
Southampton
LEVINE D F
Penzance
LIBBY D P M
London
LIVESEY H
Duphar
PIMACDONALD N
Manchester
LYDEARD S
Southampton
MAJUMDAR S K
Bexley
MCDONAGH P
Newbury
MEISNER P
London
MORIARTY K
Salford
MUMBY K
London
ORNSTEIN M
London
PEARSON A J G
Barnet
PEDLOW P R B
Stevenage

PRIOR A
Manchester
RAAB P
London
REGINALD P
London
ROBINSON J
Duphar
ROBINSON V P
Iver, Bucks.
ROGERS V
London
ROSS I N
Newark
SALTER R H
Carlisle
SAXTON D
London
SHARIF K W
Sutton Coldfield
SITARAS D A
Northolt
STEELE J W
London
SULLIVAN J
Guildford
SUTHERLAND I
London
THILLAINAYAGAM V
London
THOMAS C
London
TODD P M
London
WALSH B
Hastings
WATSON A
London
WILKINSON R W
Reading
WILLIAMS A
Edinburgh

MEDICAL RELATIONS PUBLICATIONS

CURRENT APPROACHES SERIES

Vertigo
Nutrition in the elderly (reprint April 1986)
Aspects of Vertigo
Small Bowel Disease
Alzheimer's Disease
Renal Failure
Endometrial Carcinoma
ECT
Risk/Benefits of Antidepressants
Obesity
The Biological Clock
Sleep Disorders
Childbirth as a Life Event
Sudden Cardiac Death
Neuropyschiatric Aspects of Aids

OCCASIONAL PAPERS/SUPPLEMENTS

Acquired Subglottic Stenosis in Infants(Supplement No 17) Journal
of Laryngology and Otology-November 1988

The above publications can be obtained by writing to:-
Duphar Medical Relations
Gaters Hill, West End
Southampton SO3 3JD